The HOW? & WHY? Of PUBERTY...

This book is an ideal accompaniment
to the Teens-Puberty-books:

Changes Facing-Rosie

Changes-Facing-Kian

Changes-Facing-Jai and

Changes-Facing-Caitlin

Christine Thompson-Wells
Author, Professional Educator & Independent Writer

We support Diabetes Type One & Motor Neuron Disease. 10% of the net sales will be divided equally between both charities.

Our Mission:

Every child and adult have value and is important to us; therefore, we strive through research, online education, and book publishing, to bring life-skill education to all children and all families.

For Education Packages

Please see our book website: www.how2books.com.au and Education packages, www.fullpotentialtraining.com.au
or Contact:
admin@fullpotentialtraining.com.au

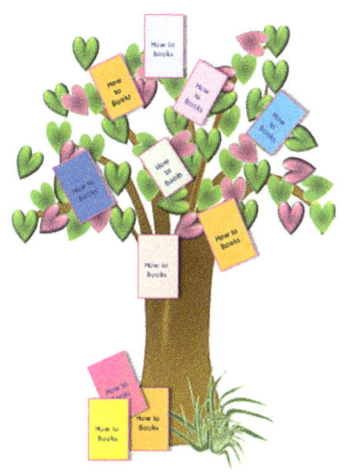

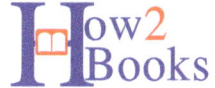

If you have purchased this book without its cover, it may be a stolen book.

Neither the publisher or the author is under any obligation to provide professional services in anyway, legal, health or in any form which is related to this book, its contents advice or otherwise.

The law and practices vary from country to country and state to state.

If legal or professional information is required, the purchaser, or the reader should seek the information privately and best suited to their particular needs, and circumstances.

This is not a medical book. It is a book developed by the publisher to open the conversation about how the human body changes when growing up.

The author and publisher specifically disclaim any liability that may be incurred from the information within this book.
All rights reserved. No part of this book, including the interior design, images, cover design, diagrams, or any intellectual property (IP), icons and photographs may be reproduced or transmitted in any form by any means (electronic, photocopying, recording or otherwise) without the prior permission of the publisher. ©

Copyright© 2022 MSI Australia
All rights reserved.

ISBN: 978-0-6451314-2-0

Published by How2Books
Under licence from MSI Ltd, Australia
Company Registration No: 96963518255
NSW, Australia

See our website: www.how2books.com.au
Or contact by email: sales@how2books.com.au
Covers and Copyright owned by MSI, Australia

MSI acknowledges the author and images, text and photographs used in this book.

Children's books

Will Jones Space Adventures & The Money Formula – Book
Will Jones Space Adventures & The Money Formula – The Play
Will Jones & The Money Formula – Educator's Resource Pack
Will Jones Space Adventures & the Zadrilian Queen – Book
Will Jones Space Adventures & The Zadrilian Queen – Play
Will Jones Space Adventures & The Zadrilian Queen – Educator's Resource Pack
There are many more Will Jones Books To Come Out
Dora Damper Makes Honey Damper Bread
Potato Pete Goes to Market
Changes Facing Rosie,
Changes Facing Kian,
Changes Facing Jai
Changes Facing Caitlin

Books For Adults

Devils In Our Food
Recipes Without Devil Additives
How To Reduce Stress – Find Your Positive Head Space
Making Cash Flow
Selling Made Easy
Know Your Destination 'Go' Learn To Drive Your Mind
The Golden Book Of Whispering Poems and many more books
Hormone, Puberty & Your Child and others

Please see our website –
www.how2books.com.au

Disclaimer

This is not a medical book and should not be used as such. The contents have been developed through observational theory and research (observational psychology). Information is also drawn from scientific literature, research and peer-reviewed research, web search and personal enquiry.

The diagrams are for information and to enhance the meaning of the written text.
Statements, information, and ideas within this book are for education purposes only. The text presented allows the reader to draw their own conclusions on the content offered.

Always consult with your doctor for possible illness or underlying illness. Christine Thompson-Wells (MSI) Australia, How2Books.com.au and Full Potential Training.com.au, cannot be held liable for any errors or omissions.

OVERVIEW

The journey and writing of the four books in the 'Changes' series for young adults, took about two years of research and writing.

Having said the above and having taught puberty education in several schools and with many young students, I knew my goal was to give the readers and students of these latest books, 'Changes', the whole picture of how the body works and how the brain also works when hormones are released, when going through puberty.

Puberty, in many instances, is not spoken about in the homes or schools, people become embarrassed when they start to hear such words as periods, testicles or other words relating to the natural workings of the human body. This embarrassment is part of an attitude that has been handed down, through many families since the Victorian era of *'being seen and not heard!'*

This attitude, can and does, get our teens into trouble as you will see in one case study, as you read through this book.

As parents' many grew up with limitations in material wealth or in homes where their parents, literally made 'something out of nothing,' – 'they made ends meet', as they always would say!

We are now living in a different and technological world; our children are bombarded with electronic devices, and the social media platforms seen on these devices. Many young adults, though their parents may have locking on their devices, are exposed to pornography, graphic images of females and males, and other mind-disturbing information, that would not normally be seen in their own home or on the devices within the family!

As parents, we can act, we can start to fight back and arm our young people with education and give them the knowledge of, 'How?' and 'Why?' of puberty. This knowledge will prepare and forewarn them; we will literally take the mystery, intrigue, smuttiness, and embarrassment out of the subject and make it an easily said and understood topic.

Once disarmed, the pornography sites and other sex exposure sites, will not have the intrigue or attraction, or the visual hold, it might have prior to the learning.

Yes, people, regardless of age, will always be inquisitive, but if viewed, the teen may look, but the attraction once shown should not hold the teen's imagination for long, the knowledge they have, will allow our teens to look but not linger, or they may show a complete lack of interest when peers are looking at these platforms.

Out of the five books, including this one for parents, this book was the most difficult to write. I have used my own experience, education and learning combined with peer reviewed academic papers, to support the information written within the book. It is needless to say, *'I am happy the journey is almost complete, though a lot of work, bringing this subject into everyday language and now written onto the paper, it leaves me with a great feeling of relief.'*

I too, hope you enjoy the journey of discovery written onto the pages. I sincerely hope your journey includes sharing your findings with your teen, and my greatest wish is, with the knowledge gained, we keep our teens safe.

Christine

CONTENT	PAGE
CHAPTER ONE Cutting to the chase	1
CHAPTER TWO A unique piece of human technology – the human brain	10
CHAPTER THREE The body's progression into adulthood	29
CHAPTER FOUR Food and drink, self-image, and social media	48
CHAPTER FIVE Let's take a closer look at hormones	67
CHAPTER SIX More about hormones – the Victorian attitude	83
CHAPTER SEVEN Your girl teen's health, and into puberty	113
CHAPTER EIGHT Your teen, the maturing body, health and wellbeing	129
CHAPTER NINE Your boy teen's health and into puberty	142
CHAPTER TEN The complex journey into adulthood – and again the Victorian attitude	157

PERSPECTIVE

A perspective comes into the book writing when I can relate to past students and the many experiences, we, (me as their teacher, and them, as the learners), my past students are the richest source of information I have in writing many of my books.

Prior to going to university here in Australia, I spent five years training as a florist in London. Floristry, is yes, about arranging flowers to make them look nice and to become a saleable object. However, what I discovered during that training was the way that emotions impact our lives and how we react to different life experiences in different ways! The flower industry, though many will not agree, is not about selling flowers, but about satisfying the human and emotional need to communicate with another person!

Communication, from the flower giving comes in the form of a wedding bouquet for the bride, though, traditionally, a bride carried a bouquet to keep evil spirits away while she made the vows with her new husband. Flowers and flower giving are indeed another language! This language is extended when we buy flowers because another person is grieving or in pain, or for celebration, the birth of a baby; flower giving at these times, allows, without words, to communicate with another human being.

During this learning, I didn't realise it at the time, I was indeed paving the way for my entrance to university, education, and psychology. So, the base for learning was floristry which triggered the questions that needed answers, 'Why do people buy flowers?' such experiences contribute to my writing.

After university, and while teaching in the United Kingdon, I experience a personal 'learning curve,' and I was surprised at the time! I was counselling and teaching young offenders at Huntercombe, Young Offenders Institution in Oxfordshire. As an educator, I had three great outcomes working and supporting these teens. Two inmates were committed to continue with their education, and that was not anything they had previously planned or spoken about, and the third, made a vow to go back to his training and work, and to *'never go back to Huntercombe...!'*

One day, I left the grounds of the prison and went to my car, my head was spinning and all that I heard my mind telling me, *'Most of these young men should not be in this place...!'*

Most of the pubertal males I was working with were good young people that had made silly or stupid mistakes and now, they have not only served their sentences, but may possibly have a criminal record for life!

Having been on the inside of the story, and teaching in mainstream education, it is remarkably easy for a teen to end up in the prison system, as the three inmates spoken about in the above!

As you read through the book, you will be introduced to a young male, now serving his time in a youth detention centre here in Australia. As I wrote this book, not only does my awareness go back to the young males in Huntercombe, but to the many young people who are locked up in prisons or detention centres here in Australia and around the world, because they have made silly mistakes!

Dare I say it, it is the adults, the education systems and most of all, the attitudes of the Victorian era that are supporting our young people to get into trouble, and these three areas in our society need positive action taken and attitudes changed.

Abuse, bullying, domestic violence, drug, narcotic and alcohol abuse, underage sexual activities, self-harm, low self-esteem, and young adults ending up in detention centres; these are just a few areas, that get our teens into trouble. If we are to reduce these above actions by males and females, pubertal education must be instigated by governments, actioned, and taught in all schools, and spoken about in every home. As I have recently heard one parent say,

'Oh, they find out all they want to know, (referring to her two teenage children), on the internet, they probably know more than I do!' Then there was a chuckle from the parent!

Such attitudes held by adults or mentors, are not only giving the wrong messages to the teens but negating their responsibility in teaching or working with their young adult to keep them safe.

This is not about religious beliefs, 'old hat' ideas or tradition, this about preparing our teens for the world that is greatly different because the world and its people are living in the twenty-first century, and never have children and teens faced the type of onslaught, of media presence, the young people of today face!

Our Priority Is To Keep Our Teens Safe

CHAPTER ONE
CUTTING TO THE CHASE

If you are a parent with either a child or children at the ages of seven to eight, you can be rest assured, the sexual hormones of your child are on the move, and change is about to happen to their body and the way they think and behave!

Of course, all children are different, they come from gene pools that have different characteristics that make a child a unique person.

Many parents are aware their child is growing up but don't really know about the hormones that make the 'growing up' happen!

I was talking to a couple recently, who knew little about hormones; now, that isn't wrong, because in general education, people are aware of puberty and talk generally about the human body and how it changes, but few, including educators, are aware of how puberty happens, and the role hormones play!

The journey of our body's hormones is not only interesting, but it can also become a journey of awareness and re-discovery.

Going back to the couple I was recently talking about and speaking to them while at my desk, they were not aware that hormones start with the growth hormone as the embryo develops, then at the eight weeks, the time the child's sex is determined, the hormone testosterone is produced in the embryo. Without testosterone within the embryo, the child would not become a male; testosterone allows the child to develop the male penis and the testicles necessary to become a baby boy! Therefore, hormones are active in us all throughout our lives.

Likewise, if we did not have the hormone, estrogen, we would not have our baby girls. It is the hormones that work within the embryo that gives us and our world population, our sons, and daughters!

It is the hormones within our bodies that make puberty happen. Regardless of any belief, attitude, ideals, cultures or upbringing, hormones will activate within the child when their timeclock says, 'Activate!' It is at this time, that the child will start to change.

Now, traditionally, it has been about eight years of age that changes start, but some research is now showing that puberty, may start in some children, as low as seven or even six years of age!

So how does, as an educator or parent introduce this sensitive subject to the child or family? This was the ten-million-dollar question. Sitting at the computer, I did a doodle and came up with my first hormone, that was the 'growth' hormone also called somatotropin. As time went on, I drew more of the first shape, in fact, I copied the same shape, time and time again, and then started dressing them up with different hats, shoes, signs and other embellishments. From that point of playing with the first shape, came the first of four books of 'Changes,' for young adults. Books introducing our children to the changes their body will be making as they grow into their teens and beyond those years.

For me, as an educator, it's a great journey because I love to play with my writing, and I want to enjoy the journey with my readers.

I'm not only a mum but have been in and out of the classroom over a forty-year period; and indeed, as I have said, *'I have taught puberty education.'* At the time of teaching the subject, I always knew there was a great chunk of information missing.

I did have the privilege of teaching two young groups of students between the ages of eight to nine, and nine- to eleven-year-old mixed classes of boys and girls. I have to say, they were the most amazing students I have ever taught, and both groups were at the same school. Not only did the transition from girl to woman and boy to man transcend during the lessons, but these children wanted to know, How? and Why? The journey of how and why, has been both fascinating and enjoyable and has answered many of my own questions.

As I have said, I started with the growth hormone, and the doodle that has now transcended into many different hormones, also how the image has been dressed to meet the different roles that hormones play within our body and brain. If we are to give children important information that they can use as a life skill builder, that information needs to have the ability to keep them safe throughout life. That information needs to be easily understood and meet their understanding at their age of learning. Children will not understand long convoluted words that have little to no connection to them at their time of learning!

Regardless of how a parent feels, your child will possibly want to walk their own path once they come to maturity. Before they take to their pathway, I see it as our responsibility, to give to them, the tools or learning that will support them as they travel the distance and into their future.

Learning about, how their body works is but one point, but in the learning, we need to incorporate the brain and its important role in the learning they do. Many parents put great emphasis on the intelligence of their child, but all learning needs to be supported by the mechanisms (goodness and nutrition) within the food they eat, or with the information they learn. Evens hormones within the body need to be fed well and kept well nourished! I will come back to this subject a bit later in the book!

Most children in the world, as with us all, are made through sexual intercourse or through invitro fertilization. It is sex, or intercourse, that keeps the human population going, and while there is sex, there will be babies born, so let's go back to these miracles of life.

As mature adults, and that means from the age of consent; the age of sexual consent, varies from state to state and country to country; each state or country has its community rules, and these rules are there for a reason, to keep people safe!

Having worked and counselled young offenders in the British prison system, it is easy to see why some young people get themselves into trouble! Having now done many years of research on the human brain and behaviour, and with the research for the four books for teens, 'Changes,' it is easy to see, without the knowledge of how their body and brain can change, young people are left, by many of us adults, to enter, if you like, 'the lion's den' of adulthood; this is not fair on these young people! After all, the adults of the world are the role models these young people grow up with!

And, so it is, it is the responsibility of us all, to give to our children the life skill information that will help to keep them safe as they navigate the sometimes-treacherous waters, into maturity!

With social media, being an active part of each young person's world, they are exposed to more misinformation than at any other time in human history. They see more actions on devices, than is sometimes healthy for the developing brain! Sometimes, they see pawn movies, and think that is what sex is all about, when it is not. Sex is about taking responsibility for the action of having sex, it is not a 'freebie' that is there for the 'lust' of the moment!

In the front of each of the children's books, there is a quotation I've taken from the British Curriculum, and I think it sums up the performance of sex for young people in a nutshell, here it is:

'*Effective RSE does not encourage early sexual experimentation. It should teach young people to understand human sexuality and to respect themselves and others. It enables young people to mature, build their confidence and self-esteem and understand the reasons for delaying sexual activity. Effective RSE also supports people, throughout life, to develop safe, fulfilling, and healthy sexual relationships, at the appropriate time.*[1]

The above words should ring true for many readers of this book, after all, as responsible parents, this is what we want for our children, and so it is, one of the reasons I have written 'Changes' for children and now, this book for the adults of the children I write for!

I have previously mentioned the human brain, and this unique piece of human technology, which works 'twenty-four seven', not only in the adult brain, but also in the maturing brains of our young adults, and our young children from within the womb, then into birth, and growing into their childhood! It is therefore, of paramount importance, that the brain is kept at the forefront of the writings within this book!

---

[1] Relationships and Puberty education (RSE) (Secondary) - GOV.UK (www.gov.uk) Extracted from 'statutory guidance Relationships Education, Relationships and Puberty education (RSE) and Health Education & Australia: https://www.scootle.edu.au

KEEPING FOCUS AND EXPANDING ON THE INFORMATION

HORMONES – Trigger puberty to start in a young person's body.

AGE – New research is suggesting that puberty may start in young people at seven to eight, but later research is suggesting, in some children, it might start as early as six years.

PUBERTY – Both the body and brain change as puberty onset increases

NOURISHMENT – Good nutritional food helps to keep the body and hormones healthy.

THE HUMAN BRAIN – Often neglected in any form of education; it is the role of the human brain, and its vital work done, that keeps the human body efficiently working and healthy.

TROUBLE – Because of the lack of education and guidance, many young people end up in trouble; some end up in youth detention centres and may eventually end up in jail. In many cases, this can be avoided, if information, in the form of education, is given at the appropriate age and with the appropriate understanding – reaching the child or teen's (learning capacity) at the time.

CHAPTER TWO
A UNIQUE PIECE OF HUMAN TECHNOLOGY – THE HUMAN BRAIN

As I have said in the last chapter, we each now, and our children, have daily access to more technology and advanced technology in our everyday lives than in human history. We, as parents are aware of this, but so too, are the drug dealers of the world, the pornography film developers, gambling companies, criminal platform builders using social media, and so, each child that has exposure to social media, and the devices that do not have controls on them, can become the victim of this, in many instances, indoctrination!

The susceptible human brain
At birth, the human brain has a lot of work ahead of it. For the next seven or so years after birth, your child's brain and the pre-frontal cortex is developing; this is known as the age of reason. At seven, the brain continues with ongoing development, but it's not mature. It takes a further eighteen years, when your child is about twenty-five, their brain becomes mature. Now, from birth to twenty-five, the brain has many tasks to learn and stages of development to go through. If one of the stages is missed, the child can

suffer in learning and gaining maturity. With such a susceptible human brain, regardless of the intelligence of the child, the brain of our adolescent sons and daughters needs protecting.

When a child is exposed to social media, many social media platforms become predators! It is the algorithm that is put into place by the developers of the platform, that allows our young people to become bullied and intimidated by this technology!

The vulnerability of the human brain
Recently, here in Australia, we have heard the sad story of Molly, a fourteen-year-old girl living in the United Kingdom, who took her life through viewing predator social media technology. So, how does this happen?

The human brain never switches off, it works while your teen sleeps, does their school learning, during play and while resting – their amazing brain continues to stay alert. Through either instinct or learnt responses, it will give warnings when danger is close and will continue to breakdown and dissect vital information.

As the teen grows, so does the brain, but not forgotten here should be the role the human mind plays with all incoming information

The maturing human brain

After years of observation, not only in the classroom, a prison institution, my own children, the children living within different neighbourhoods I have lived in; it is obvious that the outcome behaviour shown by some young people is a sign, that their brain is still maturing!

The research for the 'Changes' books just written, shows that learning and brain development need to be incorporated into everyday life building skills, both within the home and education.

While maturation of the brain is taking place, if overstimulated by the release of hormones, and possibly, the main hormones being dopamine and adrenalin, the brain enjoys the excitement of the moment. Even if a child is watching or hearing different negative and destructive information, for some reason, the brain becomes excited, therefore, releasing these hormones and possibly, other supporting hormones! Through this hormone release and once the child becomes a victim to negative and misleading information, the child may find the fascination and stimulation of the destructive information too difficult to let go and dismiss.

Algorithm codes put into some social media platforms, give the technology the information, and have the ability, to allow different 'Pop Ups' and other cues, when a child logs onto and opens a device. It is these algorithms that work with the codes that allow this technology to work. And so, we all witness the sad story of Molly who took her own life because of the intimidation of an algorithm! This type of manipulation is criminal and destructive with no moral conscience by the platform developer.

Molly's sad story is but one, there are many more unreported incidents happening daily and around the world.

The latest craze is vaping in schools. Only last week, one of my colleagues told me about her son; he's a new boy and just entered high school here in Australia! He wanted to go to the toilet during the break, or play break, as it is sometimes called. This young man, just eleven years old, went into the toilet block. There were older boys vaping in the block, he was told, *'go away, and don't tell anybody about this!'*

A single teacher, on yard or playground duty during school breaks, do not enter toilet blocks to stop these dangerous activities, and there is a good reason for this: if they do, they may be made responsible or possibly be charged with trumped up charges of sexual abuse and misconduct, they therefore, do not enter toilet blocks during school breaks!

Back to the story of the young man wanting to go to the toilet block, as the bell had rung, and without doing what his body was wanting to do, he went to his next class. During the lesson, he requested permission to go to the toilet! Having to get a pass to go to the toilet, he was told off by the teacher, for not using the facility during the break!

Again, how many children are there, not only within our own country, but around the world, experiencing this type of daily abuse? I would imagine, many, if not thousands! These dominating attitudes, as seen by the vaping activities of older boys, should be stopped, but with so many restrictions, now on teachers, it may be difficult to do!

With positive proactive action, a head teacher could direct two teachers to enter toilet blocks to share in the observation; each then, could validate the observation and give a true, and legitimate account of the inspection.

It will be difficult to break a vaping culture once established in the teen. The power with which industries can influence teens through advertising, can and does lead to health risks, and harmful behaviours.

Little do people realise, that every activity seen or experience, experienced by each person, leaves its mark on the human brain and in the mind of our young eleven-year-old; he will remember the experience for the rest of his life. Having said that, the young men vaping in the toilet block will also wear the experience!

Vaping has been proven to be a dangerous pastime. The substances used in vaping products can come from unregistered manufacturers, therefore, there is an 'open market' for many of these illegal activities!

Vaping can, and will interfere, with the development of the young prefrontal cortex brain in your child if they are doing this!

Let's leave the activity of vaping at this point and go back to the developing human brain of a child!

At the start of the journey when the ovum is met by the sperm, the journey into human life begins. It can be a somewhat treacherous life for the two cells once they have met and collaborate on their journey!

After all, they are developing a life-long relationship, that needs support to develop and mature as the journey progresses! From the journey of two separate cells, to the formulation of many takes time, energy, and determination, and surely this must be with some form of intelligence, that human life begins!

For the first twelve hours after conception, the fertilised egg remains a single cell. It takes about a further thirty hours for the cells to start to divide and multiply and a further three days for the now, berry like formation, which will continue to multiply, this by some medical professionals, is called the 'Bundle'. After the eighth or ninth day and while the multiplying of cells continues, the bundle is slowly carried down the fallopian tube, where the bundle or blastocyst, as it is also known, will bury itself into the wall of the uterus. Once in this position, the blastocyst will be nourished through the blood from the mother's blood supply.

At about five weeks into the pregnancy, the baby's brain, that may resemble a cotton thread, spinal cord and heart will develop. The baby's brain is an essential part of the central nervous system (CNS). Within this system, there are three parts that are critical for healthy development of the child, these are the:

- **Cerebrum,** which allows your child to think, remember and experience feelings. When the developing embryo wants rest or sleep, the sleep is triggered by the feeling of tiredness; tiredness is a feeling and experience!
- **Cerebellum**, this allows your child to lift their arms, legs while in the womb and later, and after birth, allows your child to run, catch a ball, and ride their bike. The cerebellum is responsible for the movement and actions needed later in life, which may include, driving

a truck, digging in the garden and other heavy work, including hanging out the washing, moving furniture or playing netball or other sports.
- **Brain stem** keeps the body alive. Its primary role is to keep the heart beating allowing the lungs to work and supports blood pressure.

And this is each the start of the life of our children, a miracle of magnificent proportion when we each stop to think about how this wonder takes place; we as parents, want the best outcomes for the children we bring into the world.

And so it is, our children, go into puberty, and if we do not prepare them mentally with quality information and education about how human beings are made, they can get into all manner of difficulties on their journey into adulthood.

With temptations all around them, many young people, if not prepared and informed, can find themselves in very real trouble.

As I have previously said, I have counselled and taught young men in the prison system. Some of these young men are not deliberately naughty or want to get into trouble, but they do!

A recent story has been told to me, he was just thirteen when he and his family moved back into town after living in very rural Australia. Some parts of Australia are so remote, they may take many days of constant driving to reach the destination! Moving back, our young man was naïve to sleek city girls and how 'street wise' some boys and girls can become when living close to, or within, major cities. The young man was not used to the, almost city life, he was now living within. He had a girlfriend, and for some reason, he and his girl split up. After the split, he had several different girlfriends, all appear to be from the same class at school!

He was popular with all the girls. He was good looking, had a country way about him, and girls seem to come looking for him.

After living in a rural area, and used to playing a lot of sport, this young man, was not familiar with the attraction he now had and how the young girls found him so appealing!

I suppose, we can assume he was naïve to the attention he was getting. With many girls appearing to line up to either go out with him, or have sex with him, he thought, he was in seventh heaven; but of course, like so many 'sweet' life journeys, this one has a bitter ending!

This young man was accused of rape, though, he may not have raped a girl, the accusation was made! Once made, the police were brought in, the young man is now facing an uncertain and immediate future!

The thought of sex, in both males and females, stimulates the human brain and body, through the release of dopamine, and adrenalin, added to this is testosterone and estrogen. Through stimulation in visual photographs, actions taken, words spoken in suggestions made, will prompt the release of dopamine, adrenalin, testosterone, estrogen, and is supported with gonadotropin; this hormone supports testosterone. This gives the penis or vagina the message, sex is about to happen!

The thoughts of the activity of sex happens in both males, and females while going into, and through puberty, into and through adulthood!

Not all young adults, after arousal, are aware that sex as the action, may take place! Children start to feel sex arousal from early ages which may be as young as six or seven years of age!

Sexual arousal is as much a part of the child growing up as any other growth and development done by the human body; it all needs to happen because it has a purpose. Nothing within the human body's natural development is done as a surplus! We have all been given, through nature and natural development, these feelings, and emotions and this is to ensure our survival and the survival of the species.

When children are exposed to early, and underage sexual activity or intercourse, it can and may do damage to the developing and, or the maturing brain.

If girls and boys, during early adolescence, have intercourse, they become mentally and highly sexually aroused.

A pubertal male has high levels of testosterone, therefore stimulation from stimulation of the flesh, through visual images, or by gesture or words spoken, will find attraction to a female of a similar age difficult to resist, so why is this? It comes back to the hormones within both the male and female working to a high capacity of response which is part of the process of puberty.

Once the experience of intercourse has happened to an underage adolescent, the hormones, I believe become overactive, possibly filling the brain of young males with all four hormones, dopamine, adrenaline, testosterone and the supporting hormone, gonadotropin, thus saturation of the brain by the hormones and continued stimulation; thus again, as stimulation increases, so do the demands by the brain for the experience!

If young underage adults are not made aware, through education, that underage sexual activity is illegal and is breaking the law, then the brain's demand for sex will be increased, thus the possible overriding of any ideas of wrongdoing, or breaking the law!

Young adolescent females, who have early sexual intercourse are also at risk of developing the hormone rush or saturation of the brain as outlined in the above.

Now, back to our young man accused of rape; naiveness on the part of our children, is a big price to pay for him and other young people who may find they are in a similar situation, and indeed their families! So where has this true incident gone wrong?

When it comes to speaking about the human body, sex and other intimate details of the human body, many parents, still have the 'Victorian' attitude, to *'be seen and not heard!'* If you are unfamiliar with this phrase, it is very much still used in many countries and communities worldwide, especially, in the United Kingdom.

By not giving our children the information about puberty and the different, and natural, demands the body makes of young people as they adjust, re-adjust, to the differences they are experiencing, we are doing a great disfavour and injustice to these people.

When I say we, it is not only the parents that are responsible for educating their children but too, the education systems we are living within. If education for this critical transition in life is not provided for our children by the schools, then many parents may face the situation our young male is facing; that is not a situation anybody wants to experience if it can be avoided! And avoided, it can be!

Many years ago, and while teaching, I chaired a Curriculum Advisory Committee, and curriculums are not easy documents to create. With my background, in this last year while writing, the 'Changes' series for children, I have gone through countless curriculum documents searching for Sex or Puberty education, there is very little, in fact nothing of substance for teachers to access. Many puberty or puberty education documents within the curriculum documents have a heading, but with little informative information for teachers when delivering the subject to their students. In one document I found, the only resource was two diagrammatic images of the female shape and genitalia and the same for the male!

So, how are teachers expected to teach such a sensitive subject, especially when so much of the information, incorporates how the human brain plays such a major part of the change's children experience when going into and through puberty?

And so, it was and is, this whole new area of research has opened, and that is joining the dots between hormones, puberty and behaviour or behavioural outcomes, and if not understood, can get so many children, young adults, and parents into trouble.

To give you some idea, of the mechanism of hormones, which is not generally understood, many disastrous life outcomes can come and do come into people's lives. Puberty is but one area of behaviour and behavioural outcomes! Behavioural outcome can also be related to women's behaviour during menopause! Women may find, they act differently during this time, some may commit crimes, and yet, prior to their hormonal upheaval, they were pillars of the community!

I too, have had experiences with wayward hormones. At the time, like many women in the population, I didn't understand hormones or what they could do within my behaviour. I was a sane mum with two children, diagnosed with premature onset of menopause, which was possibly brought on by glandular fever; I became a person I didn't recognise! It was not only how I felt, I felt very unwell, my behaviour was totally out of character with who I am! Overall, it was a disastrous experience for me and my family! As I recall, and write this information into this book, it makes me cringe!

Conditions such as low serotonin levels known as serotonin syndrome, can also change a person's behaviour; they may become depressed, withdrawn and have anxiety attacks, and yet, this relates to the hormone serotonin!

Because of so many different attitudes within many world communities, many children grow into adulthood not knowing the cause, for girls, the period she has, and for boys, the complex nature of sperm, and yet, these two basic areas of human existence are related to the work that hormones do!

Since time in memoriam, hormones have been playing their role in working with the human body, brain, and the development of the human mind.

And so it is, hormones are chemical messengers that are sent all over the human body, and sometimes the messenger transports distorted information, which in turn, sends a different message, other than that originally intended, back to the human brain, therein, the mind works with the information it has received and tries to make some common sense out of the messages!

KEEPING FOCUS AND EXPANDING ON THE INFORMATION

A MAGNIFICENT PIECE OF HUMAN TECHNOLOGY – The human brain that has taken many thousands, if not millions, of years to develop. This amazing brain, which we all have, needs to be understood and respected.

SOCIAL MEDIA - Whilst it may be good in some instances, can, as we have seen with the case of Molly, and with the combination of how the brain works, be used with devastating outcomes.

ALGORITHMS - There are at least six types of algorithms used in and on most social media pages. The defence parents have, only let a child use a device, when you can see the pages or platform the child is watching. This is going to be a difficult situation for many parents to monitor! It is either watch and patrol or limit the use and platform the child/teen is using, this may be difficult to do, but be persistent.

HORMONES – Once the sex hormones become active in your teen, their world, the world previously known to them, changes. They no longer see the world through their 'child' eyes, they are starting to mature in both body and brain; all such changes are triggered by hormones. Science is now telling us; sex hormone activation may start in some six-to seven-year-old children.

CHAPTER THREE
THE BODY'S PROGRESSION INTO ADULTHOOD

As I have mentioned, I have taught puberty education for three years and knew there was a 'gaping hole' in the information provided by the organisation I was teaching for, and the necessary information needed by the students! Again, the questions of 'How?' and 'Why?', needed to be answered, and they were not!

With any project, there must be a starting point, and so, it is, with hormones and puberty! Many people who work in the medical field know that a person who studies the behaviour and mechanisms of hormones, is called an endocrinologist, and yet, the understanding by many lay people of what an endocrinologist does, is not readily understood!

An endocrinologist has studied knowledge and experience within the human endocrine system and specialise in:

- Understanding of the human pancreas and its role in diabetes type one and two.
- Understanding of the pituitary gland and how it works at the base of the human brain. It

secretes and stores hormones which support other hormones that regulate body temperature, urine functions and other parts of the body that need to function at different times.

- Understanding of the thyroid gland, how this gland also has many roles to keep our body healthy. It is important to regulate heart rate and blood pressure, and amongst other roles, it helps to regulate human metabolism and helps children to grow and develop into adults.

  The parathyroid is responsible for regulating the amount of calcium, magnesium and phosphorus within the blood and bones of each human being.

- Understanding the ovaries and testes. These also produce hormones, which are responsible for, in females, the preparedness of the female egg as it becomes the ovum, and in males, the production of sperm.

As this is not a medical book, there is so much more to understanding the role of each hormone we have working within our bodies. Dissecting and gaining knowledge about hormones is an interesting field of science and research within the medical sphere, however, as 'mere commoners', we too, need to know about and understand how hormones can interfere with everyday life! We also need to be able to transfer this information to those members of our families interested in knowing how their body and brain works together!

Hormones play an important role in your daily living, including, going to the bathroom to use the toilet, having a shower. They also play a part when you get into your car to either go to work or pick the children up from school! So, it is important that these body messengers are kept in good order, and chiefly that is done through eating a balanced diet.

When your child goes into puberty, it is the activation of many hormones, including sex hormones that may cause havoc in the child and, from the actions or behaviours of the child, you may experience going through a hurricane that is only happening in your household!

It is not only during puberty that hormones can disrupt the events of our lives! I don't know if any woman reading this can relate to what I am about to say next, *'during menopause, because of an insecure home base, I became the hurricane going through the household, it wasn't nice for the family or myself.'*

Hormones can be both good messengers and saboteurs.

With our young people, if the body's system is thrown into chaos or is under attack through too much stress, changing life situations, experiencing negative feedback in the form of bullying at school, being continually intimidated by peers or siblings, having an insecure home base, such as parents splitting up, death or sickness of a parent, and more, that can cause upheaval in the emotional states and hormone activity in our teens!

Many young people are not aware of the journey into puberty and or adolescence, they therefore surge ahead without any forewarning of the perils that can exist without guidelines put into place!

Both young males and females, need to have free-flowing conversations with either their parents or a trusted mentor. They need to have support and references to equally, supportive people within their environment, As Romeo, 2010, has described, *'by adding to the exposure to an enriching environment during adolescence may offset many of the negative neurobehavioral and physiological consequences of early life adversity.'*

Brain development

As we all know, in recent years, there has been advancement with technology, this has given neuroscience great insight into how the human brain works within different environments and the type of reactions we all experience at different times and events in our lives. When a child goes into puberty, it is indeed a great event, it is the realisation, a child is now becoming an adult.

The brain, through physical growth and the interaction within the hormone supply, makes changes to the pre-frontal cortex. The connections between different regions within the pre-frontal cortex allows your child to think differently, this is known as 'higher order' thinking! Depending on the personality of the child and the environment where they live, they may be tempted to start taking risks. These risks may be long and short-term risks; they will also be looking at the rewards they will receive by taking that risk.

This is especially so, when many young people are looking to choose a career, many will want to know, even before they take on the training within a career structure, such as traineeship, apprenticeship, or other commitments to their time, *'how much will I get paid, if I do this?'*

As parents, we want our children to be treated fairly in the workforce, but the building of life skills should not be overlooked when young people are setting out on a journey of learning or gaining of information to enhance their future.

Within higher order thinking, your child may want more reasoning when in conversation with you, and ask, *'How?'* and *'Why?'*, they will want to know more intricate details, rather than 'just being told!'

Dual systems – becoming an adult
Within young people, the brain neurodevelopment process prepares, which is dual systems of

development, are part of the passage of, and, into puberty. This process has two to three areas of your child's life working at the same time, this is a response system to the demands of 1) remnants of childhood thinking, and behaviour, 2) entering adolescents, and 3) the adaption to that process, then preparing and living as a responsible adult!

Another area of brain maturity, is the response to risk behaviour, the, *'I dare you to do this!'* This is often seen in peer-group pressure. Because the young adult is still only part way through their brain maturity, there will be many fragments of *'doing as they are told!'* Being told by a group member to do something, they don't want to do, puts the child and their maturing brain under stress and into conflict thinking; this then releases the stress hormone cortisol!

So, in these conflicting situations, the young adult is not only coping with the natural physical and internal growth of the brain and body, the many sex hormones that are starting up, but the stress of peer, and adult pressure! This is a situation that needs to be understood by parents, educators, including those people working within school environments, the law within the state or country, government authorities and the medical profession.

Dual systems operating within the young adult's brain, may make them vulnerable to risk behaviour that leads them into trouble which may leave a damaging impression on the way they think and behave in the future.

Without clear guidance within your child's education from the child's parents and the school environment to which they attend, many children may find conflict within their thinking, even as an adult, if they do not fully understand their own behavioural outcomes when doing something wrong!

As an adult, they may still live in conflict with the way they think and behave! Accordingly, *'The dual-systems model emphasizes a developmentally normal mismatch between intense affective and behavioural reactions and motivations and limited capacity to regulate them* (Steinberg 2005).

From the moment of conception, hormones continue to play their role throughout life. If we have not enough or too many of any one hormone, our life can become chaos, and this is equally so for the young adults going into puberty and adults experiencing changes in their body and brain!

As teenagers develop, they must live and work within the dual system within their development; this can bring about many mismatches in behaviour, personality, and their own unique development into adulthood.

The human brain plays a unique role with many hormones that are released into the body's system, but some hormones are released from other parts of the body including the pancreas, liver, ovaries in females and the testes in males.

For many young people, the time of puberty can be a time of overwhelming realisation, they are becoming the adults of tomorrow! Many young adults, males more than females, can become insecure and be led into destructive actions, that under normal circumstances, they would not commit to or do. Many destructive outcomes are brought about by peer pressure, and or situations seen on social media and live media. Most teens commit offences through curiosity or through risk taking.

Because of high levels of testosterone circulating within the male's body system and brain, and the lack of life experiences, many male's commit offences or have negative outcomes to the actions they've taken because, they are stretching their mental capacity, and do not fully understand the law or penalties of the community they are living in.

While teaching and counselling young offenders, within the prison system in the United Kingdom, we would have many group discussions, and once these young men were confident with my role, they would slowly 'open up' and tell their story! A young inmate was encouraged by other group members to tell his story to me, and to the other members of the group, it went like this:

'Well, I was out with a group of mates, and I was dared to steal a moped!' A moped is a small engine bike. *'I*

did steal the bike, and I got caught, this is why I am here, Miss!'

The second story, has a funny slant, but disastrous outcomes for one of the inmate's, his story, was:

'I was walking past this house, and there was a really nice car in the driveway, a Ferrari; I looked inside and the keys were in the ignition, so I got inside the car and drove the car away; the car was a mess inside and needed a clean, so I took it, cleaned out the rubbish, gave the car a clean and took it back to the owner. When I got there to deliver the car back to the owner, the police and owner were waiting for me…! And that is why I'm in prison, Miss!'

Not only do our teens take silly actions, but there seems to be little reasoning and realisation, that a good deed can have disastrous outcomes!

There are other areas of our teens lives that can also be impacted by hormones, peer pressure, celebrity image and their impact, drug abuse, eating disorders and more!

I have spoken about social media and the irresponsible application of code and algorithms used on social media platforms that our young people can be attracted to.

The brain is a powerful tool and does what it is told to do by the owner of the brain

Few people realise that the brain is indeed an obedient servant and does exactly what it is told to do!

Our young people do not understand this fact and it is, indeed, a difficult concept to understand when first being told about this masterful tool! So, let's look at some of the areas of human action, once hormones are stimulated in the brain, and those that are driven by habit, and the demands made!

Social media – and hormones
Dopamine

I have spoken at length about the algorithm and code used by predators when they develop their media platforms. Our young teens, once mentally hooked on this media, can find it extremely difficult to release the habit of going back time, and time again to see the latest message or video! This physical drive to open the device is stimulated by dopamine. Dopamine is a necessary hormone released by the brain and is needed in many areas of the body to maintain good health and wellbeing. However, dopamine, is a stimulant and the brain enjoys being stimulated, hence, through over-stimulation, a habit is created!

Stimulation is needed in new school learning and academic achievement, taking on new sport activities and in self-achievement to meet obtainable goals. However, the brain only needs dopamine, and like so many other hormones, in moderation.

When, young people become addicted to social media, there is a dopamine rush.

Adrenaline
Like dopamine, the brain needs enough adrenaline released to keep the young adult safe. It allows your teen to stay safe as they cross the road; they will look at the traffic and pace their steps to move quickly out of the way of oncoming traffic; these actions are achieved through adrenaline being released from the teen's brain, with messages to their legs to, 'move faster!'

When a child becomes addicted to social media, they have both dopamine and adrenaline working in larger than normal amounts in the brain.

Within social media, and when viewing information that is targeted at immature teens, it is the activation of the dopamine and adrenaline hormone, and as I have said, '...this stimulation helps to create the habit within the brain of wanting to see more of what the platform is saying or has to offer...!' The viewing of destructive information becomes an addiction, which can, and does become uncontrollable for many young people.

Testosterone

Testosterone in young fourteen, fifteen-year-old males can be high, higher than in mature males in their thirties and forties having regular sex and those older males who have regular sex with mature adult females.

If, stimulation through seeing, touching, or suggestion are experienced by a young pubertal male, the testosterone levels may be increased! Remembering, the brain is an obedient servant, and if a child is not told about puberty, sex, and given the guidelines within the law, the child will not have any boundaries to work within.

Other considerations, not only with pubertal males and females, but with mature adults, both the vagina and penis have sensitive electronic nervous systems working within both.

Once a person is stimulated through the stimulation of seeing, touching, or suggestion, the messages, are sent to the brain of the person. (The human body works with fine sensitive electronic systems; this allows the brain to be responsive to different situations a person experiences in life.)

Our electronic body systems allow the messages to be sent from the sense experiencing the stimulation to the brain. For instance, the touch of a hand to another person, will give a message to the brain of, friendship, intimacy, or love. These messages are only made possible through the neuron pathways and through the electrical currents running through our bodies. It is from either the 'touch point' on the skin, as outlined above, through seeing or watching, through hearing of sounds or spoken words, that messages are sent to the brain.

Once the brain receives the message or messages, another message is sent to the responding hormone to deliver the response to the individual, as with the 'touch of a hand!'

There are millions of electronics running around our body and like a well looked after racing car, all the electronics need to perform when different signals are given to us. And so it is, with puberty, and our children, especially when they go through bodily changes and growing up.

Because our young people like to have their friends of similar ages, their friends are too, experiencing the growth and different body changes like your teen!

Learning and puberty
Because of the transitional nature of puberty, many teens can become nervous, moody or experience depression. Depression can also affect learning and learning outcomes. A young person may not understand that change is happening to their brain,

mind, and body, so keep the communication channels open and encourage talking about how your teen feels! A short, impromptu conversation can lift a mighty load from the shoulders of your child!

Estrogen

Estrogen is predominantly a female hormone, but like so many hormones, males also have a smaller amount in their bodies.

In female teens, estrogen is high when they reach the time within the menstrual cycle and the ovum is ready for conception of the male sperm! Like males, our teens can have higher levels of estrogen as they go through puberty. If there is a measure, pubertal males have high levels of testosterone around fourteen and fifteen years, our females may also have the equivalent at similar ages!

Underage sex in many states, and countries is a criminal offence, therefore, if we as adults, agree to social gatherings of these young people, they must and should always happen with strict adult supervision, there is more about this a little further on in the book!

KEEPING FOCUS AND EXPANDING ON THE INFORMATION

BRAIN DEVELOPMENT – As parents, and because our children are growing up, many adults think that young teens should be 'old enough to know better!' And yes, that is the case, but what we must not forget, though some teens look older than their age, the brain is developing and maturing, and many teens are working within the dual system, mentioned in this chapter, – they are neither a child or adult, sometimes in their behaviour, words said, and responsibilities taken!

THE BRAIN IS AN OBEDIENT SERVANT – With so many years of research and writing, the one thing that has given me more to think about, is the 'idle chatter' that some people develop in their heads. I haven't mentioned this in the chapter, but as the brain is an obedient servant, we can each mentally repeat upsetting events in our lives, like a broken record! If you give your brain permission to repeat and repeat an experience in your mind, that experience will soon become a habit. With respect to your mind, do not give permission for negative experiences to be held as an obsessive thought. If you find your teen is experiencing any of what I have written about in the above, work with them in meditation or with medical professionals to release the negative thoughts. It is not worth the price of stalling this work to be done. Many people do not act instantly on negative thought reduction and become victims within their own head, (a prison type existence begins), this will slowly overtake a person's life.

LEARNING AND PUBERTY – Regardless of different attitudes and belief systems, puberty will take place when it is the teen's time for it to happen! While the brain and body continue to grow, many teens, if not informed, can find the onset of puberty a frightening experience. Keeping communication channels open will support and encourage your young adult to speak about concerns should they arise.

CHAPTER FOUR
FOOD & DRINK, SELF IMAGE, AND SOCIAL MEDIA!

Many teens suffer with their self-image, and many can feel isolated from other teens of a similar age! If your teen is a loner, or has difficulty mixing with other young adults, encourage them to speak about how they feel. In many instances, social media adds to the insecurity that may be part of your teen's thinking!

A sensitive time
Through the movement and activation of hormones within the teen's body and brain, some young people start to put on weight during puberty! Because of so many celebrity images on social media and in the press, our young males, and females, think this is how they should look!

In many instances, it is not spelt out, *'Yes, they look like that because they are paid to look like that, and many make large incomes to look like that!'* If many of the images seen on social media looked different with natural weight and possibly their own natural features, many would not get the publicity they get, therefore many celebrities, and social image seekers, would receive a greatly reduced income!

A great number of young people are given false ideas through social media influencers, and what they say! We also need to look at the marketing of many foods and the influence of flashy food ads!

The availability of junk food
Much of the fast-food advertised is not healthy for the human body, or the systems that work within the body and brain, in fact much of the food advertised can be a poison to the human systems. Having said this, effective advertising is responsible for making food conglomerates millions and billions of dollars annually!

Yes, being sensible about eating good food will help your teenager to avoid the 'junk-food' offered and it is important, to understand the reasons for eating a healthy diet, especially, during puberty!

Become aware of what you eat
I have written many books over several years, but now I want to take you on a crash course of understanding how good, unprocessed food, works with the human body and brain. My research about food chemicals is an ongoing journey; I am always collecting information and it has become a journey that will never end,

because food chemicals by the food manufacturers are always being developed and added to their food products!

My book, 'Devils In Our Food,' is published and available in the worldwide market place of book sellers or from our website, www.how2books.com.au. So, too, are my books, Food Intelligence for Children, Food Intelligence for Young Adults, Chrissy Cupcake, and Devil Free Recipes. All the above books guide the reader into eating healthy, unprocessed food.

Eating unprocessed food, especially during puberty, will support your teen's health, support the immune system, and the hormones in the jobs they need to do and help to keep weight or obesity to a minimum.

The research and understanding you are about to discover, took almost five years of continuous work and investigation, so, here is your crash course in how good food helps your body to stay healthy, and how eating processed, over-sugared, trans fat cooked, fast food, helps to promote poor health, mood swings, obesity, and other health problems.

To begin, all the food you eat, the drinks you drink, and the air you breathe contains molecules. Good, natural food contains natural good molecules, natural water, contains natural good molecules, the healthy clean air you breathe, contains natural good molecules.

So, to teach children about molecules, I needed to develop an image that would show a child what a molecule looked like. A single molecule is three-dimensional in form and is a pyramid shape. Molecules are complex chains of information; this information can be both good and bad! When a molecule is changed to meet the requirements of the food manufacturer, this may be to make a food item look nice to eat, giving it 'eye' and sensory appeal, *('that would be great to eat, I can already feel my mouth watering...!')* and the customer will want to buy!

An altered molecule makes food last longer, change the colour or add to the flavour. Bad or altered molecules can also make 'dead' food look like healthy, fresh food; this is all in the art of food manufacturing!

Of course, some manufactured food is good to eat but it does make sense to read the food manufacturer's ingredient labels on the product.

Back to molecules, as I explain to the children and young adults I teach, good food has healthy molecules, processed food has unhealthy or bad molecules!

Here are the images I use to teach children about food molecules:
The pink is a good food molecule,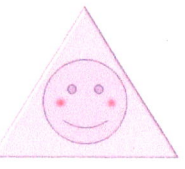
and the grey is
a nasty or bad food molecule.

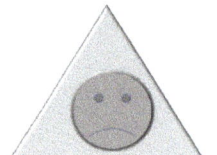

All food and drink are made up of molecules. There are four food group molecules, these are: fats, protein, carbohydrate, and alcohol. In good food the natural molecules are left intact and not manipulated like in those foods that are processed and manufactured!

Banana cube cut from fresh banana

The example I give to the children is, 'If you eat one inch or twenty-five millimetres of a banana, you will eat one hundred million of healthy molecules. If, however, you eat the same size in a piece of processed, manufactured food bar, or processed meats such as processed chicken nuggets, you may be eating one hundred million of nasty or bad food molecules!'

Imagine, a molecule is a key, and some keys don't always fit the lock!

Manufactured processed food becomes the key that needs to fit the lock within the enzymes within your gut. If the key, (the molecule), does not fit the enzymes you have in your gut, the altered and possibly 'dead' molecule has nowhere to go. It is not passed through your body in the waste you excrete when going to the bathroom to use your bowel! Therefore, that 'dead' molecule will continue to circulate in your body's system, and eventually, as more dead molecules are consumed in the dead food you eat, your body will accumulate more dead molecules that don't belong in your body; this may be the start of an obese career for you, or your family! It may also be the start of a long and destructive illness!

Little do people realise, that a great deal of processed, manufactured food, leads to malnutrition or under-nutrition! With this state of under-nourishment, the brain and body of the young person is starving, though the parents may be thinking the child has had meals, the quality and nutritional value of the food is so very poor, the body isn't receiving the goodness in minerals, proteins, correct fats, and the complexed starches the body needs, that allows it to work at its maximum potential.

Having said the above, if you find, you have given your young adult a meal, this may be a fast-food meal, and within an hour or so, they are looking for more food to eat, you will know, that your son or daughter may in fact be, undernourished because of the poor quality of the fast-food meals eaten. Malnutrition may also be evident in young people if their main food intake is from fast foods!

Back to the classroom
Having taught such a great number of children, young adults, and adults in my life, it always amazes me just how receptive young people are to receiving good,

informed, sensible information; they just want more and more of that quality information.

I have previously mentioned the incredibly intelligent children I taught while teaching puberty education to two groups of young pubertal males and females. Once getting through the information I had to teach these young people, I could see, how the lack of substance within the information I needed to deliver, was not meeting their inquisitive minds; the topic was not holding their imagination! At this point, I changed direction, and went into the 'How?' and 'Why?' of food molecules, and 'wow', we got into a great discussion about food and drink molecules, drawing the images on the chalkboard, and having instant quizzes on understanding the complexity of the food and drink they were all consuming! Literally, the walls and classroom were electric!

The teacher had never seen anything like it, but the subject linked into puberty and personal growth of these young adults, thus, the 'magic' of the lesson.

All children have great mental capacity, and so do our teens. It is up to educators and parents to find the information that 'sparks' the intelligence of each, and every child.

Self-image and the food your teen eat
Self-image plays many roles within our teen's development. They want to be accepted for who they are. Many young people keep focused, and forge ahead, and maintain a positive self-image.

For parents to support the development of a positive self-image, by speaking about becoming their 'own person' rather than that of a celebrity image, will add great compensations in your teen's life.

The lack of a positive self-image may be linked to the food and drink your teen is consuming. If your teen has weight, skin, or other health concerns, look at the food you are buying, look at the food in the refrigerator, and pantry, examine, look, and read! Look at the food ingredient labels, are those labels full of additive numbers, if so, research the additive and I suggest, once your research is done, put the food in the bin; it's not worth the packaging!

It took me well over four years to research additive numbers and some additives, you would not let some food items pass your lips, let alone swallow it!

Drugs and alcohol abuse
Many young people get caught up with consuming alcohol, and some try taking drugs, possibly thinking, they can get off the drug or drugs at any time!

I have said about the human brain being an obedient servant earlier in the book. Many young people don't realise, that just one shot of a drug can alter their brain neuron connections and over stimulate the brain to such a degree, that the one shot of a narcotic substance, can lead to an addiction!

The brain being the obedient servant that it is, once receiving the narcotic, will want more and more. If the brain does not receive what it wants, it will put on a tantrum, a tantrum just like a two-year old child.

According to Eric Berne, (Psychiatrist) each of us has three distinct parts within our personality: The Child, The Adult and The Parent. Each part of our personality plays different roles under different life conditions.

These conditions may be when you are at home, you use part of your Parent personality to interact with the children. When you are at work, you use your Adult part of your personality to give out work related orders, suggestion and ideas, and so on!

However, when, the Adult uses the Child part of the personality, there is a mismatch of actions, demands, conditions and situations!

When, narcotics or mind-altering substances are used, the Child part of the personality can become demanding and unrealistic. It is the demands of the narcotics, alcohol, or mind-altering substance, that is switching on the unrealistic demands from the individual!

The child part of the brain, which lies within the personality of each of us will shout, and scream or encourage the owner of the brain, to commit criminal offences just to get what it wants: in this instance, the narcotic for another shot!

Waiting to see a direction – florist shops and training

My first job was a traineeship in floristry, I was just fifteen at the time of starting the traineeship in London. There is very little research done that includes how the flower shop works, and indeed, I too, lived in oblivion until I continually had a running question going on inside my head: 'Why do people buy flowers?' This question led me on to university and a decade of study.

Now, you may be asking what has that got to do with drugs and alcohol?

Many years later while running my own florist shop and school, I met an eighteen-year-old woman who had been on drugs and had attended rehabilitation clinics, and indeed, was trying to keep away from drugs and the people she had been connected to, while in addiction!

As she regained her health, though each day was a struggle, I agreed to have her as a student in one of the accredited courses we were running. She was a good student, had a great creative talent and was committed to her studies.

Sadly, it was only a matter of time; she started to miss class attendance, her work wasn't handed in on time and we had no idea of how to locate her!

Weeks passed, then her parents arrived at the shop to explain what had happened! She had met up with some of the old friends and they had encouraged her to get back onto drugs; this time, there seemed to be no redemption for her.

Her parents explained, *'we have two younger children, and we cannot have her in the home while she is taking drugs!'* She was welcome at any time to go home, but under no circumstances, was she allowed to continue with her drug use.

It takes an extremely strong mind to break the habit of drug taking; the best solution, *'Don't go there in the first place!'*

Alcohol may be the start! If the immature brain receives the fantasy feelings that alcohol offers, this too, may lead to drug taking.

Alcohol is classified as a drug because of its effects on the central nervous system or (CNS). It slows the functions of the brain by reducing neural activity and inhibits vital bodily functions.

Unsupervised – a teen party
Teens love to have a party, and why not. Our teens love to be with their friends, to dance and have fun, and they especially like to do this at home!

Our young man, before he was accused of and facing a rape charge, was at a party with one adult supervising the get together! There was dancing and music and all were having fun. The adult, assuming all was well, went to bed and possibly fell asleep. The party continued, the alcohol was out and circulating, and everybody was getting drunk.

Of course, the supervising adult was possibly in a deep sleep and blissfully unaware of what was happening under his own roof and within his home! A teen couple, at the party, broke up during the night and the female made her way to our young male. With the mix of alcohol and two pubertal teens, male and female, sex was the outcome. Of course, the supervising adult was still asleep while the activities continued.

And how many more parties within our communities, and around the world go on like this? The hurt and pain experienced by the male teen, and his family are the outcome of this party!

The lack of responsibility shown by the sleeping adult, is the fault in this story which has led a young male to experience an uncertain future and possible jail sentencing!

Self-harm

Many insecure teens may start to self-harm. These young people may become lost as they transition into puberty, the change puberty brings into their life, and as the learning demands increase within education!

Many teens may think about self-harm, but not all do the act. However, some teens do self-harm because of the feelings of frustration, anger, depression, and the seemingly insurmountable challenges of their future!

When a young person feels overpowered by their daily experiences, there are ways of reducing those feelings; it is also good for our teens to remember, that harmful feelings are brought on by negative thoughts, and most challenges in life can be managed.

There are many techniques that can be used that helps our teens to work through different and difficult times, following are a few distraction ideas.

Taking the initiative – distraction ideas for your teen

- ✓ Learn to hum a tune and dance the steps to that tune.
- ✓ Hold ice cubes in the hand and keep holding them until the hands get cold; the new thoughts act as distractions to negative thoughts.
- ✓ Put a rubber band on the wrist and tell them, every time a negative thought comes into their mind, snap the band – 'ping', this is still not as destructive as self-harm, it just stings!
- ✓ Ask the teen to recite a poem that they love.

- ✓ Instead of your teen cutting or hurting the skin, draw a red line with a pen on the skin, then add a funny face, make them laugh...!
- ✓ Exercise, bounce a ball, practise shots in a netball ring – a personal ball game can work wonders and helps to create positive mental health while giving the body exercise.
- ✓ Work with your teen in deep breathing exercises, these are great to do together: breathe in through the nose, count to three, hold the oxygen for three, let the old oxygen, (now carbon dioxide) out through the mouth, then repeat again, and repeat until your teen feels relaxed. It's great for thinking, the mind, and blood.
- ✓ Ask your teen to talk to a person you trust. Guide your teen to tell your trusted person, how they feel. Your teen's life is meant to be lived, and ensure your teen, all people have a purpose.
- ✓ Encourage your teen to always have a project on the go. A project allows your teen to escape, be in their own space and allows them to be themselves.

Higher levels of cortisol may be circulating within our teen's body and brain if he or she is under stress from the school or home environment, or both! The hormone, once in freefall needs to be triggered back to normal through many of the ideas mentioned in the above, or simply take some time out and spend some quality time together.

KEEPING FOCUS AND EXPANDING ON THE INFORMATION

TRYING TO SELF-NAVIGATE PUBERTY – So many teens try to navigate their way through puberty and suddenly, the realisation, 'they are getting older!' As adults, we can help our teens. You may think, 'I'm not qualified to speak to anybody, let alone my teen, like that.' Let me tell you, we don't need qualifications to show our teen how much we love them. Giving them time and love as they walk the highway into adulthood, is a great experience for you both; the experience created is worth more than any material gains.

THE DAMAGE OF DRUGS – Many teens may think they can instantly withdraw from drug taking, even if they are only about to try it once! All brains look structurally the same or similar, but they are far from the same. We each have different neuron pathways and connections keeping us wired up; these neuron pathways relate to different parts of the body and the behaviours we exhibit. With just one drug intake, a human brain can be damaged for life!

UNSUPERVISED TEEN PARTIES – Don't be the parent who is charged with neglect or other similar charges if your teen has a party; stay alert and be ready for action if needed. It does beg the question, the teen spoken about in this book, is a real person, he is possibly naïve because of the lack of pubertal education, and his youth! However, with the consumption of alcohol, at an unsupervised home location, is not only immoral but illegal. We need to ask the question, was the sleeping parent charged with breaking the law?

CHAPTER FIVE

LET'S TAKE A CLOSER LOOK AT HORMONES

Helping our teens understand how hormones work in their bodies is what this book is all about, and I make no apologies for my hormone characters, they are part of the journey of the five books, and I think, they complement the script well. Having said that, it is important to remember the complex chemical structure of each hormone, so this is included in this chapter.

So how do we teach our teens about hormones and what they are responsible for doing in our body, and how do hormones work in the brain?

Since conception, the growth hormone has been working in our body; without this hormone, we simply would not exist! Other hormones also play important roles and many work on different timelines that only work when males and females reach certain ages and development as in puberty!

It was with the progressive images that the young people books took shape, and the necessary hormones were developed into the four books, 'Changes' for young adults.

The sole intention of hormones is to work for the good health and wellbeing of the human body.

The Growth Hormone (HGH) – Somatotropin

The growth hormone (HGH) otherwise known as somatotropin, allows the body and brain to grow, is produced in the brain's pituitary gland, and regulates height, bone density, and muscle growth. The growth hormone also regulates metabolism, builds, and repairs tissues in the brain and different bodily organs. This hormone boosts growth during adolescents, it helps to regulate body fluids, and reduces body fat by increasing bone density.

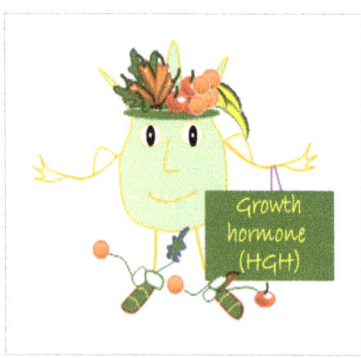

In children and young adults, the hormone is released during and within the deep sleep states. Therefore, all children and young adults need to have a regular sleeping pattern that allows their body to do the work it needs to do.

This hormone is also a peptide[2] which is responsible for cell reproduction and cell regeneration in humans and animals.

Growth Hormone chemical structure

In the above, you can see the complex structure of the hormone.

Testosterone

It may come a surprise to some people, that both males and females need to have testosterone working in their bodies. It is produced in the testes of males and in the ovaries and adrenal glands of females.

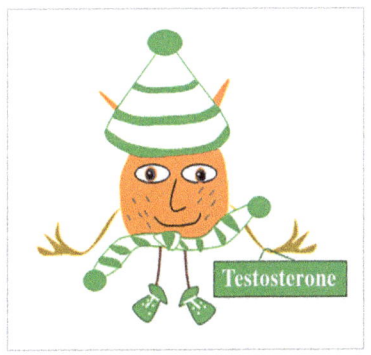

---

[2] Smaller than a protein

Testosterone is needed for the development of male sex organs. During the mother's pregnancy, testosterone helps in the development of the penis and testes in the unborn child.

During puberty, testosterone, helps the growth of hair in the armpit, around and within the pubic area; it promotes the deepening of the male voice; the development of muscle mass and strength, and works in the manufacture of sperm production.

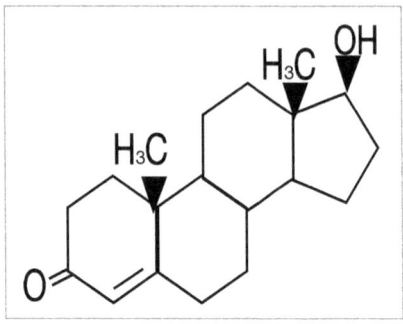

Testosterone chemical structure

Testosterone plays a key role in both males and females. Other benefits of testosterone: it aids in bone strength and helps to fight bone disorders such as osteoporosis in males and females.

Not only is testosterone responsible for hair, and muscle mass development, but it has a role to play in mood and quality of life, verbal memory, and a male's thinking ability.

In a fourteen-to-fifteen-year-old pubertal male, testosterone may increase by thirty percent and reduce as the male enters his thirties and maturity settles in.

Gonadotropin

The hormone Gonadotropin's main function is to help to control the functions within the ovaries and testes.

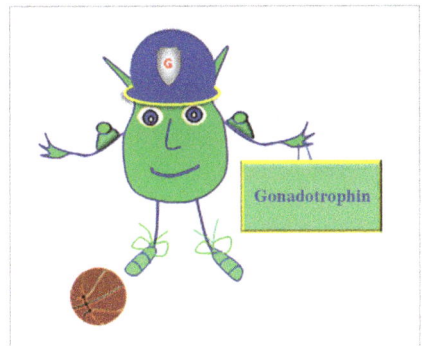

Gonadotropins are important for the regulation and proper functioning related to male and female reproduction. The main function of gonadotropins is to work with the gonads, meaning, the gonad is the sex reproductive gland in both males and females.

Gonadotropin chemical structure

Gonadotropins are made in the pituitary gland in response to other hormone stimulation in the hypothalamus. The process of production is carried out by the hypothalamus pituitary gonad axis.

There are three areas of gonadotropins, which again consist of two peptide chains, remembering that a peptide is smaller than a hormone, and in this instance, works to support both testosterone and estrogen. Like testosterone, males too, make estrogen but in smaller quantities than females!

Estrogen

Estrogen is the name given to a group of hormone compounds. It is a main hormone and is essential to the female menstrual cycle which can go from twenty-one to thirty-five days.

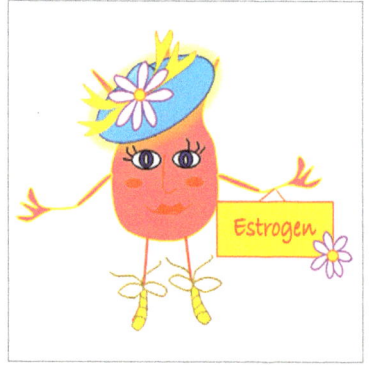

Estrogen helps a girl's body to mature. It also helps to make the bones stronger, and to keep the heart and brain healthy.

Women and girls have three types of hormones that work within the reproductive menstrual cycle:

estrogen, estradiol, and estriol. Estrogen binds together estradiol, and estriol. Both males and females have this hormone.

In biologically male bodies, estrogen is needed to balance testosterone.

Estrogen also helps to protect the brain; it helps with our memory and in some of the fine jobs it helps the fine muscles in our fingers to work! Such jobs as decorating a cake or when we are doing fine craft projects, such as painting as in art; it helps when females put on their makeup!

When both males and females work on electrical projects, it helps to keep their hands steady when they are welding fine wires and so estrogen is very important in our everyday lives.

Estrogen chemical structure

Estrogen also helps when a female's body is ready to make a baby, and in the growth of male sperm, so it has many vital jobs to do...!'

Estrone

Estrone can store estrogen and helps with female development and plays a part in female reproductive health. Like most hormones, these

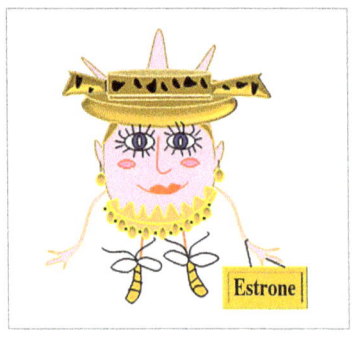

work with your body's clock. Many hormones can be sensitive to your body changes. An example may be seen with severe dieting without medical advice or guidance, these actions may put our teen's hormone activity out of balance.

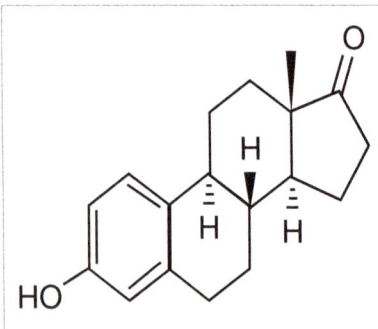

Estrone chemical structure

Estrone can be synthesized from cholesterol and secreted from the gonads. With diagnostic strength, estrone and estriol perform weaker activities than estrogen.

The female body can convert estrone into estrogen when the body needs extra estrogen for different jobs it must perform.

Estrone helps support female sexual function and development. In females, mood swings, fatigue, low or irregular bleeding may be a symptom of low estrone.

Because estrone forms and is stored in the fatty tissue of the body, extra estrone can lead to obesity and weight gain. If you have concerns, please seek medical advice.

Estriol

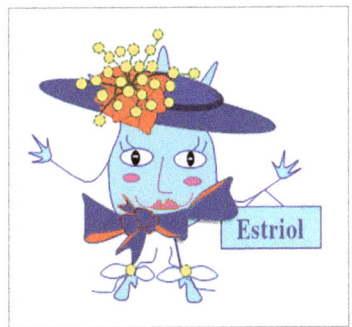

Estriol, like estrone, and estradiol, helps the female body to grow and become ready for womanhood. Like so many hormones, it too, works with its own clock and will click into gear when it receives certain messages from the brain of our teens and the female population.

Research is revealing, estriol appears to offer a wide range of health benefits to several health conditions, some of which include rheumatoid arthritis, multiple sclerosis, thyroiditis, and psoriasis. Please speak to a qualified health practitioner if this has raised issues with you.

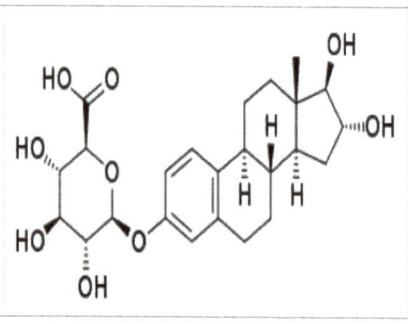

Estriol chemical structure

Estradiol

Estradiol is also a female hormone, produced primarily in the female ovaries.

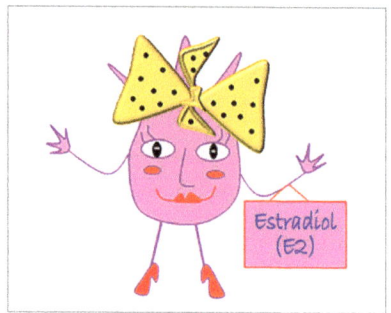

Estradiol levels can vary depending on the phase of the female menstrual cycle. It is also involved with the adjustment of the female reproductive cycles. During puberty it supports the development of breasts, widening of the hips and the fat distribution within the body. It also helps the female body in the maintenance of the reproductive tissue within the uterus and the breasts.

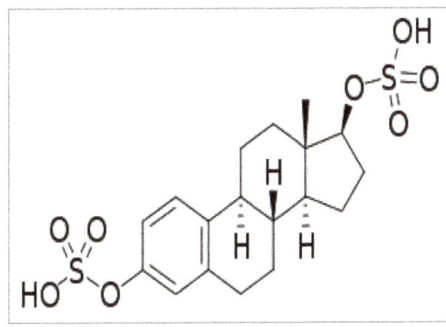
Estradiol chemical structure

Its positive contribution also helps with maintaining healthy body tissue, bone, fat, skin, liver, and the human brain.

Males also produce lower levels of estradiol in their body which helps to support male health.

Progesterone

Progesterone is released from the female ovaries. It helps when females start to have their periods, and in the body's control of the menstrual cycle. It, like many other hormones, has many functions.

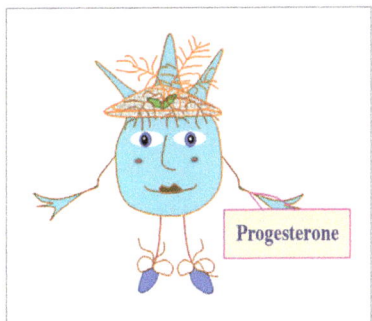

Before fertilisation, it supports the function of human sperm in the migration through the female vaginal tract after intercourse.

Progesterone plays a key role in breast development and supports the maturation of breasts (mammary glands) during pregnancy which allows for lactation to develop allowing the mother to breastfeed her infant.

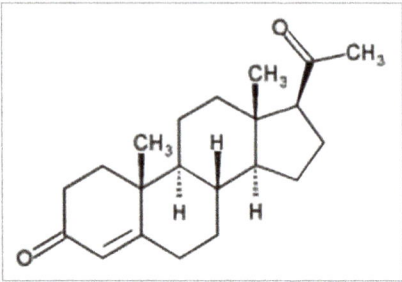
Progesterone chemical structure

Studies have shown that progesterone supports normal neurone and brain development, and if damaged, the hormone has a protective effect on brain damaged tissue.

Ghrelin

Identified in the nineteen nineties, it's also known as lenomorelin. It is produced in the human gut and lets us know when we are hungry.

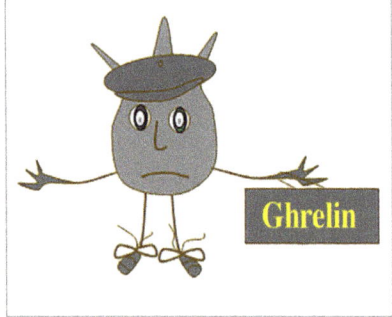

It sends a message from the gut to the brain saying, 'I'm hungry.' The message is received by the hypothalamus in the brain. The hypothalamus helps in the regulation of many hormones, and ghrelin is just one!

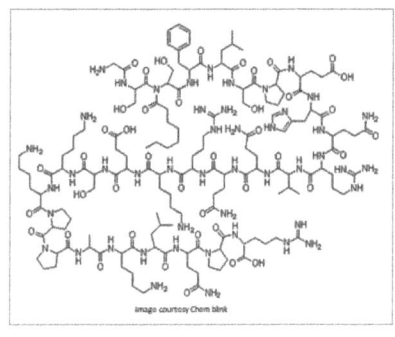
Ghrelin chemical structure

Ghrelin's main function is to increase appetite and encourages eating more food than is possibly necessary for a healthy body to function. The nature of the hormone may encourage eating more calorie foods which are stored in the body's fat, thus increasing weight if the extra calories are not used in work or exercise!

The higher levels of ghrelin, the hungrier you become! Woven into the demands of this hormone's work, maybe the eating habits of junk or processed food.

The ghrelin hormone can give us a great deal of information about the obesity crisis the world is currently facing! By working with your body, understanding the food and drink you consume and how your body's hormones work, will help you to understand the different processes and demands puberty can put into our teen's lives.

KEEPING FOCUS AND EXPANDING ON THE INFORMATION

THE COMPLEXITY OF HORMONES – OUR BOY TEENS – We are only just reaching the 'tip of the iceberg' when it comes to speaking about hormones! From a baby to a child, and we now know, that males have high levels of testosterone at birth, and this reduces as the male grows into his boyhood, only to reintroduce itself at about seven years of age. As a young male enters his pubertal years, he may experience many erections and the release of sperm from the penis. This is a natural function of the body that helps to keep the penis and sperm healthy. Like so many of the body's natural functions, once puberty starts, our teens need our support.

THE COMPLEXITY OF HORMONES – OUR GIRL TEENS – As I taught and spoke to many of the young people sitting in front of me, when I asked the question, *'How many of you suffer with headaches?'* The number of hands that raised would reach about ninety-eight percent! It would appear, that many young people do suffer with headaches at the onset of puberty, now identified as Puberty Migraines. Our pubertal girls may have these headaches about two weeks before a period begins. Other research is suggesting, low estrogen levels may also cause severe headaches in both males and females.

Stress may be causing some of these headaches, add to this, the movement of hormones and the body's readjustment to the changes, then add school stress, peer pressure, social media, too much screen time, eating junk or too much processed food, or disruptions in family life, such as family arguments, families splitting up, and divorce, may be the combination that will make living in the twenty-first century, a difficult time to be a teenager!

Reducing stress can be done by eating a whole, good food, natural diet, (a diet without junk, processed food), playing sport and other positive body exercises will support the hormonal level to a natural balance and re-adjust in the pubertal teen.

CHAPTER SIX

MORE ABOUT HORMONES -THE VICTORIAN ATTITUDE!

The story of our hormones goes on, and this is the world our teens need to navigate if they are to stay safe, and well. Staying safe, includes the way that the demands of both the male and female's body work during puberty and into adulthood!

The reason we are all here, breathing and working in our global societies, is through our parents having sex and making babies! Or through, with technology, invitro fertilization!

Ovulation

Now is the time to face reality, according to professor and obstetrician, Melissa Simon, of the University of Northwestern Chicago, *'A woman can ovulate without having her period!'* The first and youngest female known to give birth was a five and half year-old child, living in Peru in 1939. This child was raped and gave birth to a baby boy. This case of lack of identification of the rapist is unlikely today, when DNA samples of heritage and identity can be taken, whereas, as you know, this technology was not available in 1939!

We all know that puberty is part of growing up, and in earlier times, when survival of the species was paramount to human survival, females, possibly, had babies at younger ages than is now part of our law!

Old hat – Victorian attitudes make our teens vulnerable

We no longer live in the Victorian era, and it is time to take a mature and adult approach to this subject of puberty.

Having taught psychology over several years, it was not until I taught puberty education, that I became aware of the lack of informative information available to our younger people, teens, teachers, and indeed, their parents. It is the hangover from the Victorian era that makes this topic so unpalatable and uncomfortable to many people, and after all, it is just an attitude that is owned by many people that keeps the old mindset, *'seen and not heard,'* alive, and all the time, this attitude owned by many people reading this book, puts our children into danger!

Testing you out!
When I walk into a classroom, to break down the misinformation, I give the children my name and then say proudly: 'Penis', 'Vagina', 'Periods', 'Testicles', 'Sperm', 'Breasts', and 'Nipples!' I also add other proper words like 'Erection', 'Testes' and explain what is meant by some of the words, especially words like periods, this gets the embarrassment out of the way. Sometimes, I repeat the words; this touch of classroom magic takes the shyness and embarrassment out of the students, and they are ready to learn the real lesson.

Now, I test you to say the words, say them loudly and repeat them, 'Penis', 'Vagina', 'Periods', 'Testicles', 'Sperm', 'Breasts', 'Nipples', 'Erection', and 'Testes'. Now, repeat them to your children. Get them used to hearing the words, it will work wonders for introducing 'open communication' about puberty and, indeed, possibly their own experiences if they are pubertal teenagers!

The pubertal male and female
The pubertal male and female, at the ages of thirteen, fourteen and possibly up to eighteen, have higher levels of both testosterone and estrogen and other

supporting hormones running around through their body and brain. If our children and teens aren't made aware of this hormone activity, they can and do get into serious trouble.

Adolescence – the rapid development of the brain, body, and different behaviours

Puberty is a time of great change for our teens, especially with their brain and body development and sexual maturation leading to reproduction. During this time, there are major changes to the central nervous system (CNS), and the teens psychosocial behaviour. Neuroscience has made great progress in the study of the maturing brain of teenagers; this maturation process, and as I have said previously, continues until their mid-twenties.

Your teen will want to become more of their own individual and will develop and adopt new peer groups. This transition from teenager to adult is a necessary process into the adult world. Accordingly, *'A range of social determinants of health arise in adolescence, with peers, schools, and eventually the workplace becoming strong determinants of health and well-being as the influence of the family wanes!'* (Viner and others 2012)

Puberty or adrenarche

Puberty or adrenarche, is the early stage of sexual maturation, and as mentioned, in some instances, may start in children as young as six years of age. So how does puberty start?

Research and further investigation are contributing to our knowledge of this subject and is suggesting that adrenal glands may contribute to the ongoing brain development and the associated behaviours, that may get some young people into trouble. It is this mismatch of chemistry, neuron connections, or lack of connections, behavioural actions and outcomes as identified in the dual systems information spoken of earlier in the book. From the research undergone, and accordingly, *'Adrenarche has few phenotypic[3] signs in most children, but increasing evidence indicates that adrenal androgens[4] may contribute to the structural and functional development of the brain and associated behaviours in adolescence.'* (Whittle and others 2015). The increasing information should help to reduce the

---

[3] Phenotypic: a characteristic or trait.
[4] Androgens help start puberty and play a role in reproductive health and body development.

antiquated ideas of the Victorian attitude of being *'seen and not heard!'*

Adrenarche, or early puberty onset needs to be understood by all adults, not excluding any one person because of 'old hat' ideas, beliefs, 'old wives' tales', traditional out-of-date thinking, family belief structures, or doctrines.

Not only are there changes in the body's system, but there is the development of pubic hair, body odour, oily skin, and the awareness of sexual attraction to other people of a similar age or, in some instances, older or younger people! There is also the awareness of increased sexual drive, (libido), and desire. These are all natural desires, that need to be managed and controlled by the owner of the body. This jolt into adulthood, may lead to mismatches of behaviour, though, the child may still be, (and look like a child), and in the 'child body,' the brain and hormones may be years ahead of the developing child; this presence of self, can, and does, lead to confusion for the teen.

None of what has been outlined in the above are dirty or wrong. They are after all, the natural maturation of the human body and brain and should be respected as that.

Back to hormones

Hormones make life happen, without hormones, we would not be here breathing, working, loving, experiencing, achieving, and having families, so we have a lot to thank hormones for.

Serotonin

We have spoken at great length about many of the hormones that circulate through our body and brain

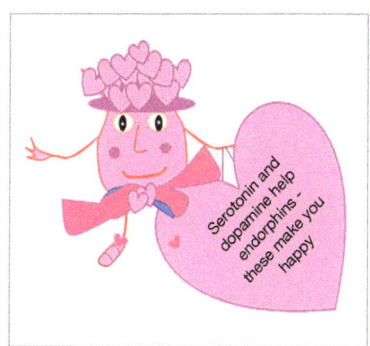

and have mentioned both testosterone and estrogen hormones. Other hormones also play a vital role in keeping us alive and healthy. Serotonin is needed to perform bowel movements and helps to keep the intestine healthy. Serotonin is not only a hormone, like all hormones, is a chemical messenger that carries messages between nerve cells. It helps with mood adjustment, developing regular sleep patterns, bone health, helps wounds or cut skin to heal, supports your digestive system, helps with learning and academic attainment, but it too, helps with libido, or sexual drive, and desire. When serotonin is balanced and working in the human body, it also helps with 'happiness' feelings.

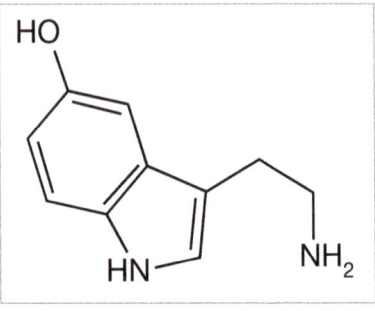

Serotonin chemical structure

When there is reduced serotonin, we can feel lonely or unhappy.

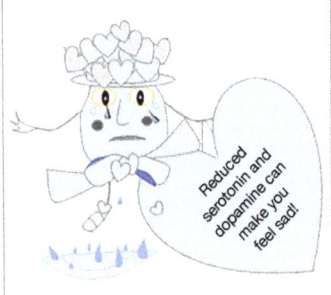

Reduced serotonin can lead to problems in mental health, depression, anxiety, mood swings, suicidal behaviour, panic disorders, digestive, and sleep problems, phobias, and, or schizophrenia.

We can all support the good health of our hormones by eating a balanced and healthy diet. Some suggested foods for serotonin balance, include salmon, eggs, cheese, turkey, pineapples, fresh nuts, oats, and seeds.

Do not eat fast take away, deep fried trans fats processed, over-sugared foods if you want healthy hormones; that diet will give you excess weight, build up cholesterol and add to health problems. Please see my book, Devils In Our Food.

Oxytocin

Oxytocin, or the 'love hormone' in so many instances is not understood!

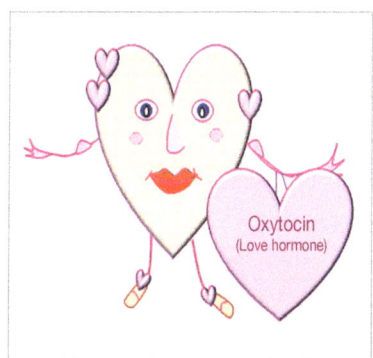

I'm sure we all have times when we think, 'we are in love!' This may be more so, when we are in our teens and going into or through puberty, or indeed later in life…!

Our teens are no different, when it comes to their emotions, they don't have the experiences the older generations have in managing feelings or emotions; this then becomes a dilemma, can be a painful experience, or a steep learning curve for them!

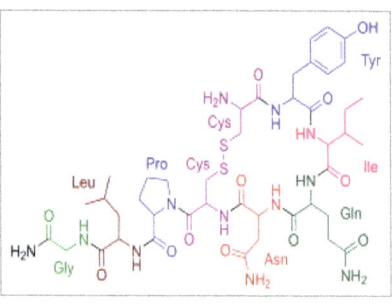

Oxytocin chemical structure

Low oxytocin levels

If a male or female has unrequited love, and if the feelings are not managed, this can lead to other emotional states and the body's reaction, which include,

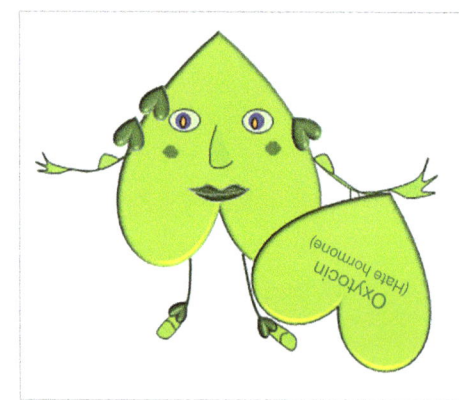

- ➤ stress
- ➤ poor self-esteem
- ➤ lack of sleeping properly
- ➤ isolation and
- ➤ lack of confidence.

Other outcomes of this include limited touching, and feelings of abandonment.

Remedies for this situation include,

- ➢ go out with other people, you don't have to be in love with a person to enjoy their company.
- ➢ hobbies and projects are great to have when life seems like hell on the other side of the front door!
- ➢ reconnect with old friends, and importantly, reconnect with family members.

All these activities help to boost oxytocin. Above all else, eat a healthy diet.

Cortisol

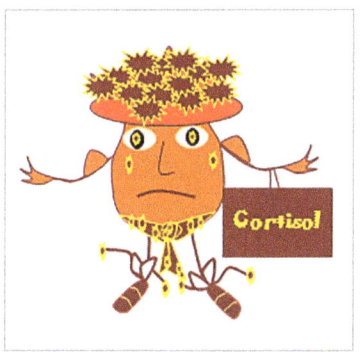

Cortisol is sometimes referred to as the stress hormone; it is a naturally occurring hormone which is made by the adrenal gland. The hormone is used throughout the body but is controlled by the hypothalamus. It controls both the body temperature and our emotional activity.

There are three main functions for cortisol working with the hypothalamus, the pituitary gland, and adrenal glands; the three configurations create the hypothalamus-pituitary-adrenal axis or (HPA).

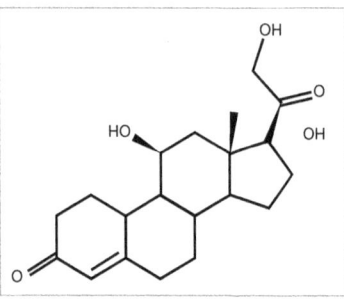

Cortisol chemical structure

Most cells and cell receptors in the human body contain and work with cortisol. Cortisol is important to maintain your metabolism and/or sugar levels, lowering inflammation, the salt and water balance of the body, memory formation, foetal development in the unborn child, and blood pressure. It also helps in the digestion of your food and manages how your body works to separate the protein, fat, or carbohydrate in the food you eat. So, it is not only a stress hormone, but it is an important hormone that helps your body to stay healthy.

Cortisol levels fluctuate daily, they are high in the morning when you wake and lessen during the day. If, however, you experience stress during the day, your body will release more cortisol, this is called the 'stress-response' we each can experience when facing difficult situations. This is also known as the 'fight or flight' response. To keep the subject simple, when we experience a threatening situation, the body's sympathetic nervous system (CNS) tells the adrenal gland to release the hormones epinephrine (adrenaline) and norepinephrine. This release of hormones gives the signal for your heart rate to increase, increasing blood floods to your muscles and prompts a fast reaction by your limbs and other areas, including words said, and actions taken.

To give an example, under stressful conditions, we may experience the inability to eat, this may be during relationship breakups, emotional upheaval as in children facing difficult life situations and other areas of 'real life' experiences.

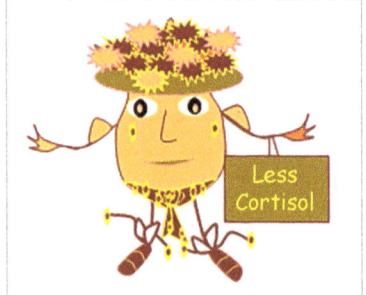

During such times, the body may also shut down the autonomic functions to conserve energy; this shutdown allows the body to use more resources, which may include the digestion of your food, hence, the need to be aware, that steps need to be taken to reduce the amount of cortisol running through your body and brain, this can instantly be done through deep breathing exercises as described on page 64.

Like all hormones, cortisol is in the body to help you, or your teen survive painful, hurtful, or frightening situations; keeping cortisol to a normal level is beneficial for several reasons,

1. Too much stress and cortisol release, zaps energy from your body and leaves the body depleted of any goodness gained from the good food eaten.

2. Too much stress and cortisol release, leads to the inability to think clearly to do daily jobs like driving the car or truck, sitting, and successfully completing examinations and other necessary jobs needing to be done.
3. Too much stress and cortisol release can reduce the immune system leaving the body susceptible to infection.
4. Too much stress and cortisol release, leads to premature aging and future long-term sickness and other negative outcomes, many of which can be avoided, by thinking proactively rather than reactively about situations, and the later conditions that may develop!

Adrenaline

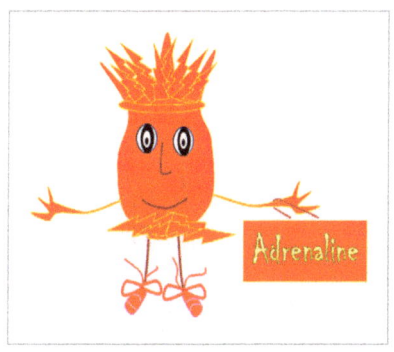

It is not only our teens that suffer with too much adrenaline flowing in and around their body and brain, but also parents. If we are to support our young people as the transition into adulthood, we too, need to know and work with our body and the body's systems.

Parents, carers, teachers, and many other people who work in our communities worry about our young people, and our teenagers. This worry, can and does lead to mature adults having an 'adrenaline rush!' So, what is adrenaline?

So far, I have spoken about many hormones, but really, there are so many, over fifty, and I'm only mentioning a few in this book!

Our adrenaline glands sit on top of the kidneys and work almost remotely until they are needed in an emergency or in times of facing different stress situations. Adrenaline is also called epinephrine and works with the adrenaline gland and connections to some neurons. The adrenal gland is responsible for making many hormones, including, cortisol, aldosterone, adrenaline, and

Adrenaline chemical structure

noradrenaline. The adrenaline gland is controlled by the pituitary gland in the brain.

Adrenaline, as mentioned is also known as a 'fight or flight' hormone' and is a necessary hormone to keep us safe. If we or our teen perceive a threatening situation, a message is sent from the amygdala in the brain, through the circuit back to the hypothalamus, the hypothalamus is known as the command centre of the brain. The hypothalamus communicates with the rest of the body through the autonomic nervous system (ANS), which works within the body's electrical circuits, to the adrenal medulla. When the adrenal glands receive the message, a signal is sent through the body's electrical circuits in the blood stream, to the adrenaline gland which sits on top of the kidney. From there a message is sent to the pancreas to release more glucose into the blood stream, this gives the body the energy to act.

When our teens get into trouble, there are many emotional processes that take over and each hormone related to the body and brain situation will kick in. We don't have to tell the hormonal system to do its job, it does it intuitively and works for our wellbeing.

The process is complicated

The system automatically goes into gear:

1. adrenaline sends or attaches to receptors on the liver cells to break down sugar molecules.
2. this allows for binding of receptors on muscle cells in the lungs, this makes us breathe quickly.
3. this stimulates the heart to beat faster.
4. the contraction and system allow blood to be directed towards major muscle groups, as in our legs, which allows us to move quickly and out of danger.
5. contracting muscle cells below the skin encourage perspiration.
6. further messages are sent to the pancreas which inhibits insulin production. Under normal everyday conditions, insulin production regulates the amount of glucose allowed into the blood stream of the body to do everyday chores, however, under stress, insulin production is inhibited giving the body a greater volume of adrenaline. Therefore, too much adrenaline experienced over longer periods of time can be damaging to the human system.

Many of our teens and younger adults experience sleepless nights, this can be caused by incidents at school, because of threats made to them if they speak or tell anybody about what they saw, or experienced! At this point, I draw your attention back to Chapter Two when an eleven-year-old boy wanted to use the toilets during the break. The older boys were vaping in the toilet block, when the younger boy wanted to use the facility, he was told, *'Go away, and don't tell anybody about what you have seen!'*

Our eleven-year-old, would have experienced stress at not being able to do the body's natural function of releasing waste from his body, but then further being told off by the teacher for requesting to go to the toilet during the next lesson time!

Our body's ability to create extra adrenaline in times of danger is a survival instinct handed down from our ancestors, but we need to know more about how it works. Some signs to look for:

- nervous tension or irritability
- dilated pupils
- rapid heart rate and breathing

- sweating
- heightened senses showing reluctance to go to school or other institutions, including primary, secondary school or college.

If you notice these signs, STOP, look, and listen to what you are witnessing!

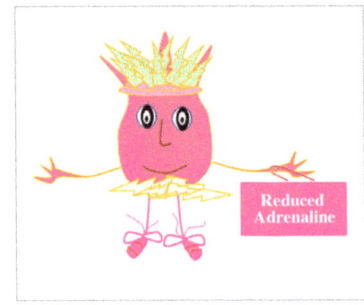

Knowing how to control adrenaline

- Encourage your teen to try meditation, if you practise this method of relaxation encourage them to join you.
- Encourage regular exercise like sports of all types, especially those where they can go and shoot a goal.
- Encourage regular talks or family nights. Turn off televisions, tablets, devices, including the mobile phone.
- Importantly, turn off all devices an hour or earlier before bed. It is the stimulation of the blue light from Smartphones that emits a blue light enabling you to see the screen during

sunlight. The Smartphone does not want to go to sleep like the human brain. The blue light restricts natural melatonin to be released from the brain, therefore stopping natural sleep occurring.
- ➢ Reduce or suggest a change of diet from a junk-food and drink diet to a healthy food and drink without additives. Some additives work as stimulants and should be avoided before sleep.
- ➢ Encourage deep breathing exercises as written on page 64.

The above will help to reduce adrenaline and contribute to sleeping well.

Dopamine

Is known as the party hormone. It is good to party, and we all need to do this activity every now and again!

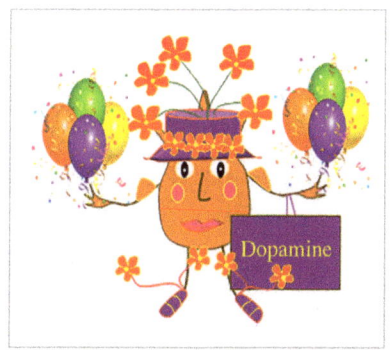

However, when there are high levels of dopamine in the brain, the brain is telling you to party, this is not always a good idea. Many party feelings or 'wants' can be brought on through drug or alcohol abuse! Having said that, dopamine is needed in many areas of everyday life. It helps with the following:

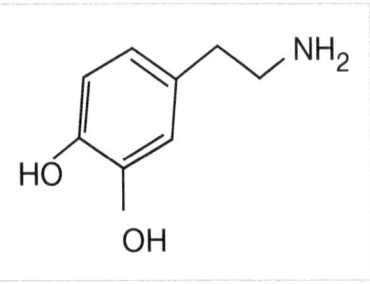

Dopamine chemical structure

> It helps with focus and attention to different jobs, developed skills such as driving a car, and operating machinery.
> It helps our teens when they set about to study for examinations in their learning and motivation.
> It also contributes to mood and sleep.
> Dopamine assists with control of nausea or vomiting and how we process pain when it is experienced.
> It assists with blood vessel and kidney function and movement.
> It helps with your heartrate.

> It may also be responsible for determining the length of time information stays in the short-term, or long-term memory.

Dopamine, like so many hormones, is known as a chemical messenger and plays a vital role in sending messages between nerve cells.

It lets us know how we feel and when we feel pleasure, it may want more pleasure than is healthy for us to have. This includes the stimulation our teens experience when their brains, through over stimulation from drugs, early, before consenting age, sexual activity, and alcohol. When any of the above happen, the young brain is not mature, therefore, the over stimulation may create many health problems, problems from within the law and problems that may be classed as illegal activities for our young teens.

Drugs such as cocaine gives a fast increase of dopamine to the brain once inhaled or injected into the body's system. That then satisfies the reward system in the brain, however, once the threshold is raised, (as with underage sex, and other brain stimulants or activities), the individual will want more of the drug or activity. During this time, the body will make less natural dopamine, this may lead to mood swings, aggressive behaviour, contribute to either short or long-term poor health outcomes!

Low dopamine

Once the brain is over-stimulated from the hormones of dopamine and adrenaline, the craving for more may become insatiable for the brain. At this point, the habit has been created and to retrieve a normal balance of hormone activity, it may take many years of clinical therapy.

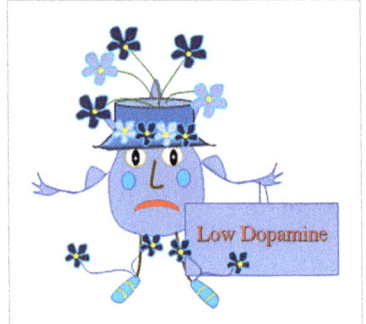

Once the drug, activity as mentioned in underage sex, or narcotic[5] taking stops, it may lead low levels of dopamine being released from the brain.

---

[5] Narcotics are any drugs that dull the senses and commonly become addictive after prolonged use.

Performing physical activities like walking, swimming, ball games, are all good exercises, that naturally raise dopamine levels. Returning to a healthy diet, as with all good hormone treatment, eating a healthy diet will also increase natural dopamine to be released from the brain. Such foods as:

- Eggs
- Almonds
- Chicken
- Beef
- Avocados
- Bananas
- Egg plant
- Citrus fruits and
- Tomatoes

Will help to balance out and normalise dopamine levels.

Low dopamine may lead to:

- Mental health issues such as depression.
- ADHD and ADD: If you are a parent with concerns about your child, their school performance, and negative behaviours, check the food you buy; (look for additives and other

nasties that may be incorporated in the ingredients panel on the packaging)
- ➢ Lack of motivation/s.
- ➢ Too tired to even try!
- ➢ Cannot concentrate on topics or quickly lose interest in the topic or what is being said!
- ➢ A feeling of hopelessness.
- ➢ Moodiness or anxiety attacks or issues.
- ➢ Trouble sleeping or disturbed sleep.

If your teen is experiencing any of the above, please seek professional medical advice.

Melatonin

Melatonin is made in the pineal gland, a small pea-sized gland, found in the middle of the human mid-brain in the brain.

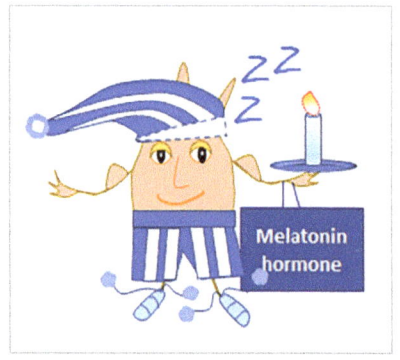

It works as a stimulant to the body and tells us when to sleep or when to wake up! This hormone works in response to darkness.

The hormone works with your teen's body clock and the forces of night and day. Once evening starts to descend, the body clock kicks in, and your teen will start to feel sleepy. Melatonin levels, in healthy people are elevated for around twelve hours, allowing people to work, study, play or do hobbies. With such activities in the day, a normal melatonin level will support people to have a good night's sleep!

Melatonin has many roles, it not only regulates the sleep cycle; in females, it plays a role in the menstruation cycle. Research is showing that young people, during puberty, may have low melatonin levels.

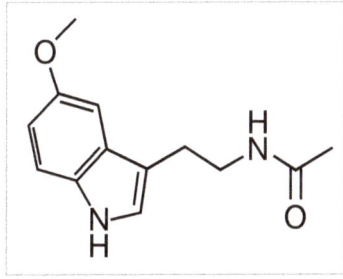

Melatonin chemical structure

In reduced melatonin levels, it may cause mood swings, disruption in sleep patterns, depression and other health conditions.

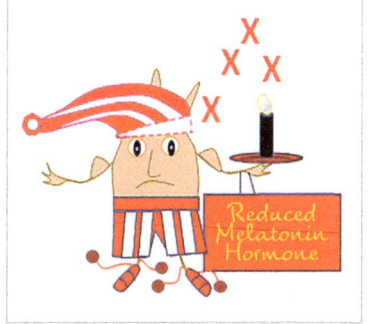

However, too much melatonin can cause headaches, drowsiness, nausea, and dizziness.

Like all hormonal levels, each needs to be balanced in the body. By eating a balanced diet that is rich in fruit, vegetables, nuts, and protein, including a variety of fruits: bananas, berries, cherries, oranges, pineapple, corn, asparagus, tomatoes, olives, broccoli, peanuts, sunflower seeds, flaxseed, and mustard seeds also include in the diet, chicken, eggs, fish, cheese and some whole grain, complex carbohydrate, such as whole grain breads. All these foods help to increase your melatonin level.

KEEPING FOCUS AND EXPANDING ON THE INFORMATION

OVULATIION – There are some ideas that a girl needs to have a period to become pregnant! As research is showing, the female ovum may become mature and be sitting in the fallopian tube at an early age, therefore, ovulation has taken place.

THE ROLE OF OUR BODY'S HORMONES – It is with great length that we have brought our hormones activities into the subject of puberty. Regardless of being a male or female, it takes many hormones, to work with your teen's body clock to make puberty happen! Accordingly, the teen's body clock will work when it is ready and is a direct force within the natural development of your child.

THE VICTORIAN ATTITUDE – How many people have suffered because of this outdated attitude? More importantly, in the twenty-first century, we need to understand the lack of education received by our teens and the preparedness they require that will support them as they enter puberty.

A HEALTHY DIET – This topic cannot be stressed enough! In my research for my book, 'Devils In Our Food,' it took four long years of reading and researching food additives. In the beginning, there were just over three hundred additives listed on the Australian government website, the number may still be the same! Having said that, with international food research now taking place, the latest research reveals a staggering ten thousand food additives are now going into the world food supply chain. Every poisonous additive added to food, will make someone, somewhere sick, this may develop into long-term illness for some!

Large food conglomerates are adding extra processed sugar, processed salt, processed trans fats and poisonous additives to many children's foods and drinks

We need accountability from food manufacturers of the food ingredients that are now added to everyday bought food. Transparency of food ingredients are being camouflaged by glitzy television and media advertising, which includes people looking healthy and active and yet, many breakfast cereals have unhealthy amounts of processed salt, processed sugar, unhealthy additives, and trans-fat, all of which contribute to poor hormone performance in our children and adults, thus, making for an extremely unhealthy world population in the future!

The addition of food additives in everyday bought food will make a sick world population, while making food conglomerates wealthy – this needs to STOP.

CHAPTER SEVEN

YOUR GIRL TEEN'S HEALTH AND INTO PUBERTY

Puberty is a natural and healthy process for all young females. At the point of bodily changes, becoming a woman, while still in a child's body, may be a major change, and if not made aware, can be a daunting experience in a young female's life. I have said many times, as parents, we do not or cannot predict when this change will happen! Therefore, by working with the young teen's books for girls', 'Changes', the journey of explanation of how a female's body changes can be easier for parents, or other adults, to explain how female change happens. By going step-by-step, with a young person, and through the information held within the books, it will open the conversation, not intimidate, or frighten your teen, and it will become a comfortable experience for you all.

The early and first stage of puberty - adrenarche

I have mentioned adrenarche in the previous chapter but will now expand on that time in your teen's life. The first signs of puberty with our female, is when 'budding' of the breasts takes place, this is usually about two years before her periods start. Budding is the development of the female breasts. During this time, the breast area may become tender, or seem hot to touch. After one of my lessons when teaching puberty education, a young student wanted to talk to me after the lesson. She was a little distressed, and I asked, '...*do you want to talk?*' She replied, '*Yes.*' We then had our conversation. The ten-year-old, was a small child by comparison to the rest of her class. As we spoke, she explained about the tenderness in her breasts. It hurt her to run, and play sport, her breasts were hot, and she could feel the changes within their development taking place! As we spoke, I asked, '...*have you spoken to your mother about this?*' She replied, '*No*'. I suggested she do so!

During the conversation, I also suggested using a cooling cream that would help to make her skin feel nice and it would help to support the stretching of the skin that was taking place. The following week, I asked the student if she had mentioned her concerns to her mother, and she had. It was a relief, as her teacher, to hear that she now had the courage, through the interaction within the puberty lesson, and the points she had learnt, to step up, and reach out to her mum.

The reason for the hotness, itchiness of the skin is the development of breast tissue taking place beneath the skin, thus the movement and activation of the female hormones.

It is recommended, to wear a supporting brassiere, or supporting tank top, may help our teen while her breasts are developing during budding.

As hormone movement takes place, hormones, including estrogen, and the associated hormones that work within the female body, turn our child into the woman she will become.

Taking it step-by-step
Stage one and as your teen grows into womanhood

By taking the initiative and speaking to your young adult about the growth they will go through in the next few years, prepares them with good and informed information;

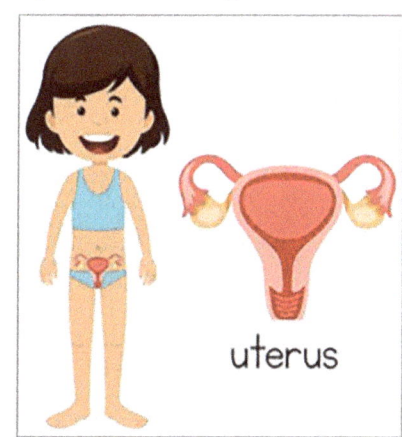

Courtesy, Pixabay image

you are forearming, and forewarning her of the changes her body will make.

By taking this action, you will alleviate any hidden and mysterious ideas they may be thinking about, or indeed, worried about!

In the diagram below, you can see there is no thickening of the walls of the uterus. This may be seen as a resting stage for our girl's body.

This diagram shows the stage after a period and during the time the uterus is resting and while the body's hormonal system prepares for the next period. During this time, our young females can feel extremely well. This is a great time for all girls; they don't have to think of anything apart from doing the normal everyday things they did before their periods started. Having said that, it does take responsibility and management for our daughters to manage their

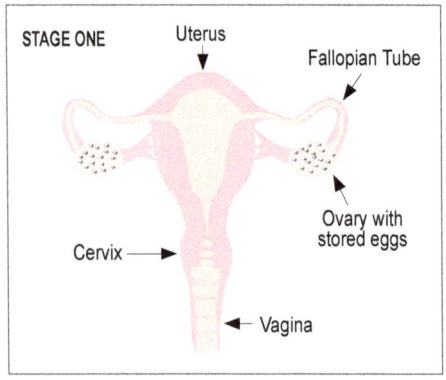

menstrual cycles, so please support them as they learn these new life conditions and demands.

Stage two

At this point, and if not made aware of how her body is changing, your daughter may feel or be irritable.

In this diagram, you can see how the wall of the uterus is thickening, and the mature egg (ovum) from the fallopian tube, has moved forward and is about to enter the uterus.

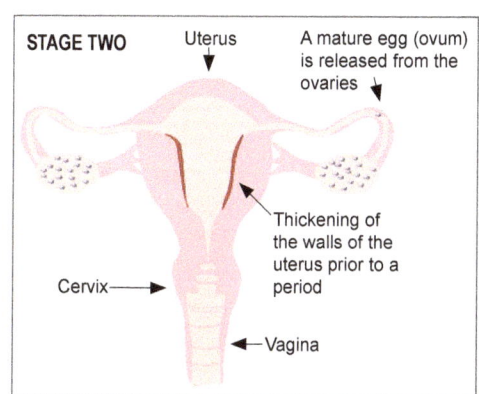

The egg or ovum is the largest cell in the human body and carries a great deal of genetic information.

This activity and movement all comes back to the hormone clock working in our daughter's body. Having said the above, by making your young female aware of what is happening within her body, she will start to understand the reasons why she feels like she does!

Stage Three

In this stage, the girl's body is getting ready for the next period. At times, our girls can feel unwell, they may have headaches and become a little lethargic.

If this is so, regular exercise and some sport can pay dividends when keeping the young body healthy.

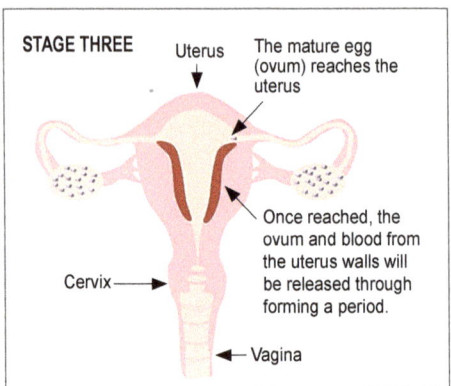

Though our teen may crave, sugary, fast food at this time, explain the benefits of eating good, natural food. For example, natural fruit and yogurt, even add a spoonful of honey to satisfy the taste buds in the mouth and the craving for something sweet to eat! The benefit of this food is that the natural food molecules are still intact and not altered through manufacturing and fast-food production. Though the food is natural, excess, can still add weight, so please be aware! If seconds are wanted, encourage your girl to wait twenty minutes, and then if she is still hungry, have a second helping!

Each girl's period cycle may be slightly different, so as you work with your daughter, do not become alarmed if her periods are at different times. During the early years of going into puberty, your daughter's body, though maturing, is not mature; she is still developing. Her body is also coping with the new demands that nature is imposing on her.

Stage Four
And finally, the day comes, when the period arrives. This is also known as menses, this signal lets you know her uterus is maturing, but her body is still in the early stages of maturation and should be respected as such.

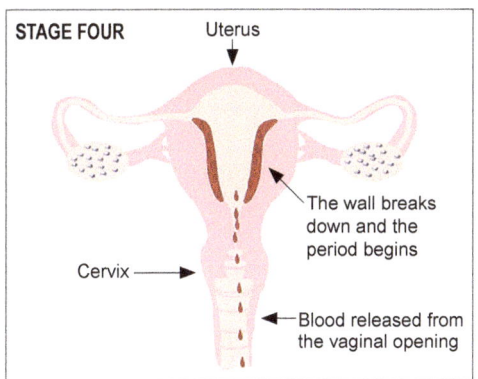

It should be a joyous occasion, as our girls, enter this new stage of life.

The first period can be light in colour and only last a short time. As I have said, all girls are different, and each girl's body will work to its own natural rhythm.

Once the period has finished, the cycle begins again. There is no mystery or intrigue to how the human body works in both males and females; the more openness to the subject, the less stress is placed on young people making the natural life journey into adulthood.

The female's body cycle

Over the course of twenty-one to thirty-five days; the usual number of days are variable but usually, about twenty-eight, the inner walls of the uterus start to thicken with extra blood. Over this time, a mature egg (ovum) is released from the ovary and travels down the fallopian tube. If the egg is not used to make a baby, it will travel into the uterus, the extra blood on the walls of the uterus will be released, creating a period.

The Female Menstrual Cycle

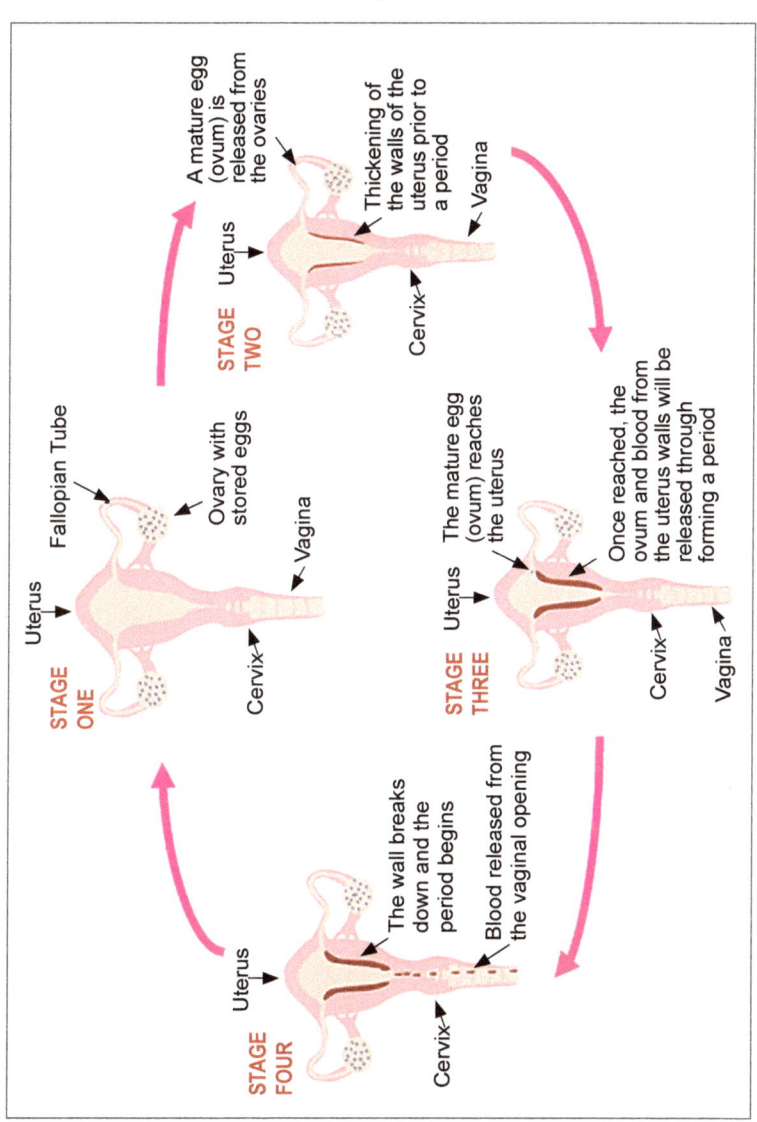

Once the period is over, the cycle begins again; the cycle will continue until the female reaches menopause.

Knowing the cycle

Having the knowledge that their body is doing what it is meant to do, can reduce stress, anxiety and worry from our daughter's life. It is worth the investment of time to enjoy the journey into womanhood with her.

The second phase of puberty – gonadarche

It is during this stage that our daughters become sexually mature. If guidelines, information, and education are not in place, it may leave a young female vulnerable to persuasion and into early sexual activities and sexual pursuits. Though the girl has reached this stage of reproduction, her physical body is not ready to carry a baby, she is still growing, and her bones are still maturing! It is at this phase, the pubic bone starts to develop strength, but is still not fully developed or may be lacking in strength to support a full-term pregnancy. The pelvic bone, sometimes called the pubic mound is part of the female anatomy and plays a vital role in supporting the growing child during pregnancy.

A young girl's body does not have the strength in either the uterus, bone structure or body strength that an older pregnant female has.

Underage sex

Though immature, both the penis and vagina are extremely sensitive areas of the human body. The activation of early sexual activities highlights the sensitivity of the human electronic systems in both the penis and vagina, thus adding to the arousal within both young people.

By taking part in early sexual activities and remembering that each person's sexual drive is driven by hormones; over-stimulation of hormones, when too young, are not healthy activities for a developing and maturing brain in any young person. I have discussed the release of the hormone dopamine earlier in this book, and the release of too much dopamine and adrenaline during sexual acts, can and may over-stimulate the immature brain, leading the young person to want more sexual activity.

From observations

Once the stimulation of too early, sexual activity, and depending on the young adult's physiology, once the brain is overstimulated, the person loses interest in schoolwork and other learning to be done. The concentration span loses objectivity and concentrates on the feelings gained from the sex they're having. This leads to lack of learning at a critical time in life.

Once stimulated, the brain can be an extremely demanding servant held within our heads. Sex drive by all people has different levels of participation, but if sexual acts happen too early in a young person's life, it can lead to people becoming mentally scarred and lead to insecure relationships later in life.

From page seven, I repeat:

'Effective RSE does not encourage early sexual experimentation. It should teach young people to understand human sexuality and to respect themselves and others. It enables young people to mature, build their confidence and self-esteem and understand the reasons for delaying sexual activity. Effective RSE also supports people, throughout life, to develop safe, fulfilling, and healthy sexual relationships, at the appropriate time.'[6]

---

[6] Relationships and Puberty education (RSE) (Secondary) - GOV.UK (www.gov.uk) Extracted from 'statutory guidance Relationships Education, Relationships and Puberty education (RSE) and Health Education & Australia: https://www.scootle.edu.au

Early sexual activity and the law

Earlier in the book, I have spoken about a young fourteen – to fifteen-year-old pubertal male who was facing criminal charges because he had sex with several girls in his class at school. Both the girls and boy appear to have little to no puberty education, and both seem to have been willing to perform the act. I have also spoken about unrequited love; no one person, knows what goes on in another person's head! Though sex may have been consensual at the time, or under the influence of alcohol or drugs, with all parties participating, with unrequited love, one girl, can, and may cry, 'rape!'

The story appears to have a consensual overtone, with all knowing that each female was having sex with this young male. Once the allegation of rape was made, the police had to be notified and criminal charges were brought against the male.

If underage sexual activities are taking place, and with few guidelines, and the lack of education, many girls and boys may find themselves in a similar situation and breaking the law!

Maturity of the human body

There appears to be a two-to-four-year window from the onset of puberty to the maturation of the sexual system within each of us!

Gonadotropins and the production of gonadal steroids continue to stimulate more growth and development across all organs of the body, and the central nervous system (CNS). With gonadotropins and other hormones doing their jobs, body fat, muscle development, and bone growth will continue to work as our daughters continue with the pubertal journey.

With this added growth happening, it is an extremely good reason to eat a healthy and balanced diet of whole food which will in turn support the body, hormone activity, brain maturity, and the immune system.

For health benefits, do not eat processed, trans fat or over-sugared food that will not support the body.

KEEPING FOCUS AND EXPANDING ON THE INFORMATION

ADRENARCHE – At adrenarche our girls' bodies and brains start the extensive changes that start the journey of puberty and into womanhood. I also highlighted my conversation with a young female after teaching a session on puberty education. The knowledge she gained during the lesson, allowed her, with confidence, to speak to her mother and the discomfort she was experiencing during breast budding. Once the threshold is broken, many conversations can begin with both our young females and males.

GONADARCHE – During this time, the enlargement of the scrotum in males is the first and immediate sign that puberty is well underway. In females, the ovaries increase their production of sex steroids. There is an increase in the production of testosterone in males and estrogen in females. Without guidelines in place, conversations in the home or education in the schools, this can be the time when under-age sexual activities take place, and our teens can end up in trouble!

RESEARCH AND ONGOING INVESTIGATION – Through research, investigation and ongoing case studies, many teens performing underage sexual activities can become emotionally scarred. This hurt may take a lifetime to repair. Another area of underage sexual activities can be seen when males or females carry the burden of forced sex, or rape. As my research continued, an older woman told me about her story. Her story took place in the sixties where she was training to become a nurse. At the time, she was about sixteen. The story goes, '*...the other nurses held me down, while he, the male, raped me..!*' It was a story that needed to be told. There are many stories like this that still need to be heard...!

CHAPTER EIGHT

YOUR TEEN, HER MATURING BODY, HEALTH, AND WELLBEING

As with life, so many experiences we have are about the process. Puberty is a process and the human evolution into maturity. It is a time of growth, understanding and development, not only of the body, but of the all-important and vital human brain.

So many parents put a great emphasis on the intelligence of their child, but few take into consideration, the diet the child eats, the hormone and hormone production going on inside the child's body and brain, and the necessary processes, that must work in the body's system, to enable puberty to begin and go through the maturation stages.

Most females, not all, want to have a baby at some time in their life, this once again is a process.

The sperm journey

For a female to produce a child, a mature egg (ovum) is released from the ovary and travels into the fallopian tube, this is Stage One. If fertilisation doesn't take place, the ovum will continue its journey until it reaches the uterus and once there, the unfertilised ovum will be released which forms part of the female period, we have seen how this happens in Chapter Seven.

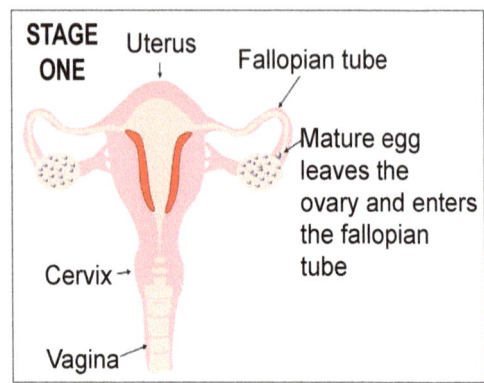

After sexual intercourse, as can be seen in Stage Two, the sperm travels up the female vagina. Sexual intercourse should be about two consenting people of the appropriate age, coming together because they want to share and love each other!'

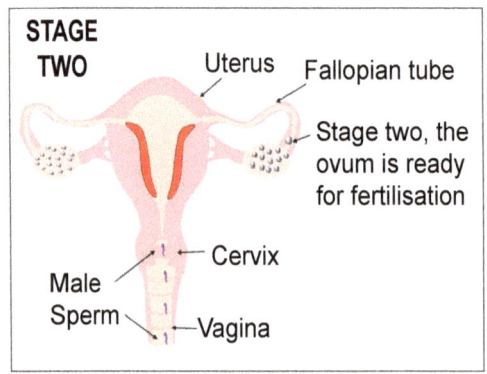

So many times, sex is seen as just and action without responsibility or feelings! If this is the case, there may be a need to re-examine personal values, and respect for each other!

Fertilisation

Fertilisation is a complicated process for the human body to achieve!'

When ejaculation of sperm from the male body takes place, many millions of sperm are released at one ejaculation! Accordingly, from the World Health Organisation, (WHO), '15 million sperm, that's around 75 million, if the man ejaculates 5ml of semen.'

So, what is semen?
Sperm is made in the testes of the male and many million are made in each male every day, some quickly die while some survive and become part of the male ejaculation process. This is a healthy process for the male as it helps to keep the male body and penis healthy.

In Stage Two, and during intercourse, and at ejaculation, sperm are released from the penis, and travel up the female vagina. Prior to ejaculation, and after leaving the testes, sperm do not have the ability to travel long distances unless they have a resting place on the journey to ejaculation. Once sperm reach the prostate gland within the male's body, they are revived by a combination of carbohydrate, sugar-based liquids including fructose, protein and catecholamines which include adrenaline, noradrenaline, and dopamine, which contribute to the hormone supply of the sperm. The combination of sugars, protein, and hormones within the semen, allow the sperm to travel to their destination.

It is the activation of many of the male and female hormones within both people participating in intercourse, that make intercourse happen. Without hormones, we would stop breeding, and humans would come to a stand-still and literally, to a dead-end!

In Stage Three of the sperm journey, the sperm meet the ovum of the female, and if a healthy connection is made, pregnancy will happen.

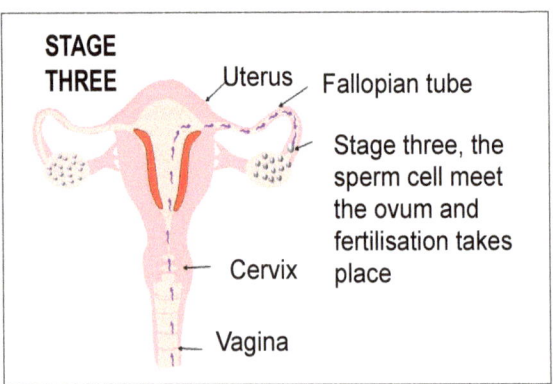

The four phases of fertilisation

Phase One

In phase one, the strongest sperm reaches the egg and is ready to fertilise the ovum. The outer rim of the female egg has a mucus edging, this helps to protect and keep the egg safe as it goes on the journey within the female body.

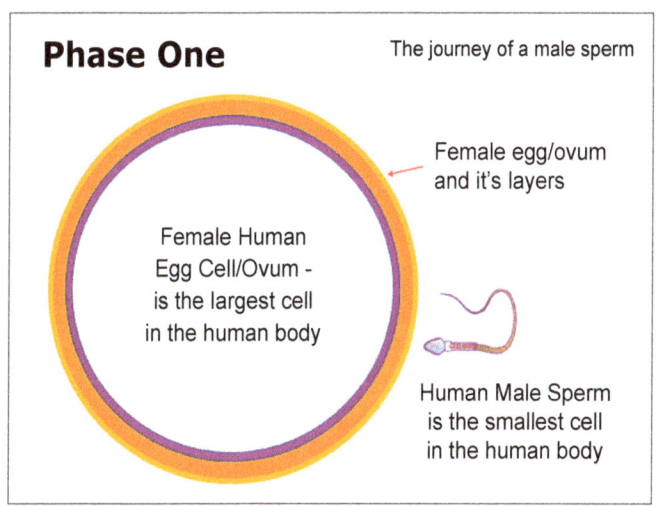

Phase Two

Within the second phase, the sperm loses its tail and the head of the sperm, which has an enzyme edge, as can be seen in purple in the following diagram. The enzyme allows the head to burrow through the mucus and outer rim of the female ovum, this allows fertilization to take place.

The mitochondria of the sperm body are absorbed into the development of cells as they divide and multiply.

It is the mitochondria handed down through the mother's genome system that the child inherits; this information allows the child to have hereditary characteristics within its own genetic makeup.

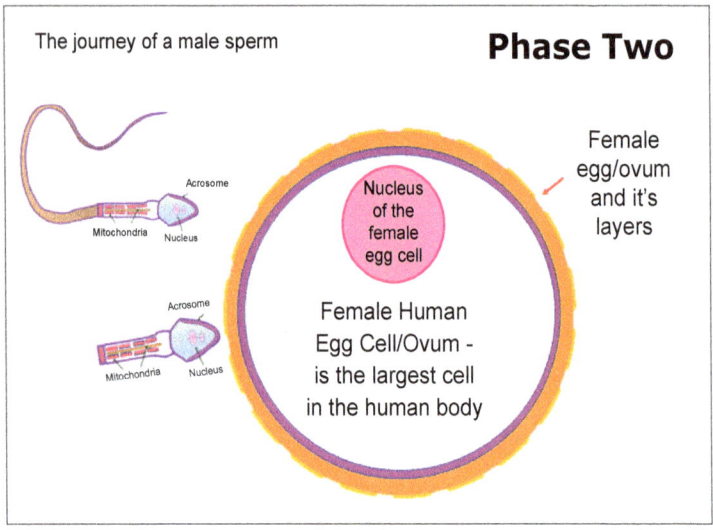

Phase Three

Within the head of the sperm lies the nucleus. The female ovum has its own nucleus, once both nuclei meet, this then becomes a power engine that work as one.

It all seems very simple in the above diagrams, but we should not become flippant about the transferring of genetic information that is taking place at every millisecond of the development of the cells, they are indeed, simply wonders of magnitude.

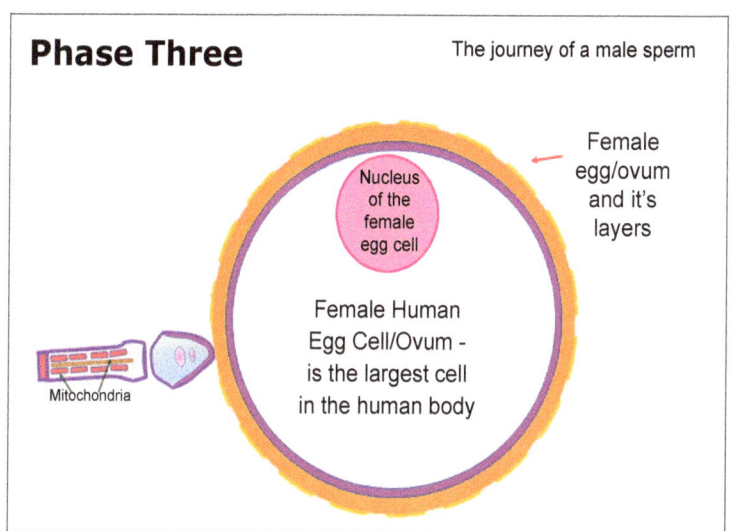

Phase Four

Both nuclei have connected and now the coming together to continue to divide and multiply. Once the multiplying of cells in the fallopian tube has taken place, the bundle is ready to move down to the uterus!

There is little to no security for the fertilised cells. For a healthy baby to be born, each stage of the journey must happen with the correct number of cells dividing and multiplying, and this needs to be done at the right time in the correct sequence!

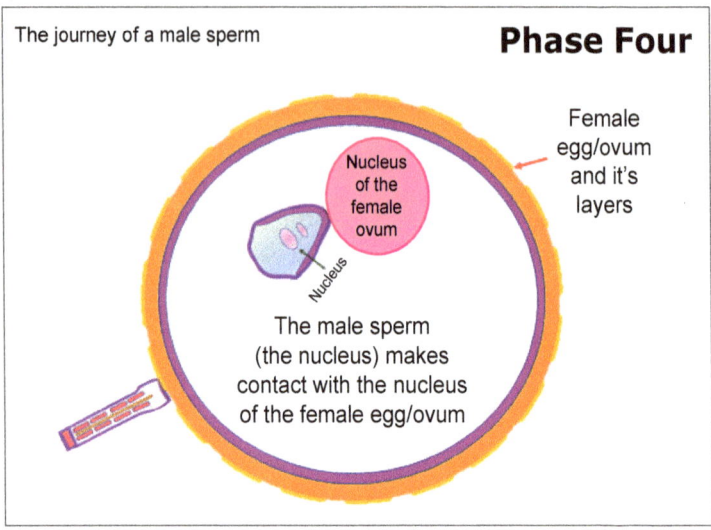

Once the cells have made their connection, they work as one in the creation of the child.

Activation and connection of two human cells

In this diagram, the male sperm and female ovum have connected. As seen in the previously spoken about phases, the sperm has penetrated the outer rim of the ovum, allowing the pregnancy to proceed. Once the two cells, (the sperm and ovum) are as one, the one cell divides into two.

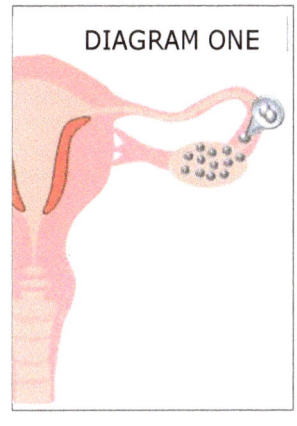

DIAGRAM ONE

At the start of fertilisation, the cells will continue to divide and multiply while in the fallopian tube, until the numbers are sufficient to allow them to form a bundle. (In some medical circles, the bundle is referred to as the blastocyst.) The number of cells in a bundle is still in discussion by medical researchers!

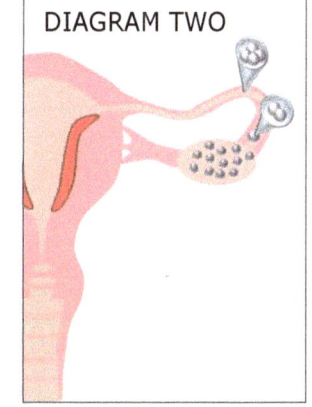

DIAGRAM TWO

In the early stages, the bundle may resemble the appearance of a raspberry. In diagram two, the division of cells continues.

The dividing and multiplying, of cells can take several days, and all the time, we must remember, these cells may become a baby.

For a healthy pregnancy to continue, the fertilised ovum needs to travel and attach itself to the wall of the uterus...!

REINFORCING THE JOURNEY

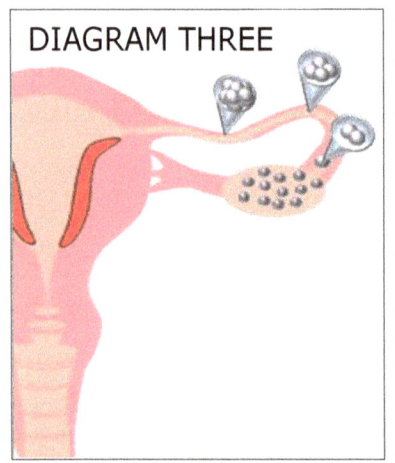

In diagram three, the cells continue to divide and multiply.

An embryo becomes a foetus after eight weeks after conception...!

For the healthy development of the bundle, the mother needs to feel secure, have the correct amount of rest, eat a healthy, sustainable diet of fresh food containing the correct fats, complex carbohydrates, unadulterated fats (natural fats), and healthy quantities of water.

In the following diagram, you can see how the bundle, has moved, and is attached to the side of the uterus!

Not all bundles or fertilised human cells survive!'

In Diagram four, the bundle roles down the fallopian tube and connects to the wall of the female uterus.

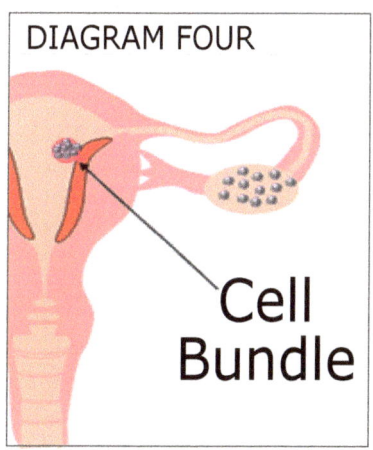

DIAGRAM FOUR

Cell Bundle

Once the connection is made, the mother's blood supply will feed into the bundle allowing the pregnancy to continue.

KEEPING FOCUS AND EXPANDING ON THE INFORMATION

SEXUAL ACTIVITY – HOW IT HAPPENS – Many teens become caught up in early sexual activity. This activity happens because the brain and body, through thousands of years of development and modification, are programmed to produce babies. Sex, and intercourse ensures the survival of the species. We are now at the stage of 'How?' and 'Why?' Intercourse is a natural part of human activity, and as I have written, it should happen, at the appropriate age and when two people care about the wellbeing of each other. Early sexual activity in young males and females, over stimulates the brain. The brain is the command centre within us all. It is however, learning to work with the brain that is the powerhouse within every human being. It controls, the thoughts we have, the words we speak and the actions we each take. The brain, if not controlled, will want instant gratification, and early sexual activity is just that; it is a command from the brain to have fun and to enjoy the moment!

EDUCATION – EARLY INTERVENTION THE 'HOW?' AND 'WHY?' - Early intervention through education has many benefits. Not only do our teens learn about how their body and brain work when going into puberty, but they can develop forward thinking, this type of maturity will only come about through the education adults transfer to the children and young adults. Forward and careful thinking encourages our teens to control their behaviour, this gives many benefits to our societies and communities. It will reduce domestic violence, drug, alcohol and gambling addictions, abuse of children and young people, crime on many levels, and other blights that contaminate our own and world societies.

PUBERTY – THE AGE OF RESPONSIBILITIES – It is difficult to comprehend that puberty may start in some children as early as six years of age. It is the activation of hormones that start to make the changes in your child. Regardless of the age, a child is still a child! Each child will go through similar hormonal activation stages at their body and brain's appropriate age!

THE OVUM AND FERTILIZATION – GIVING THE TEEN THE INFORMATION – We have seen in this last chapter how the fertilisation happens once the sperm penetrates the ovum. Once fertilization takes place, there is little protection for the cells and the developing bundle, soon to become a baby; therefore, there is a great responsibility on teens, when they participate in underage sex! Teens cannot and will not understand their responsibilities unless they receive the appropriate education at the appropriate age. It is therefore suggested, by preparing your teen, while still a child, with the knowledge about how their body, (and to mention, at a suitable age, how their brain, are growing), and they too, will start to grow, and see things differently!

RESPONSIBILITY AND MATURATION – I have taught many children and young adults, and it always amazes me just how caring many of these young people are. They care about their future, the future populations, the planet, its animals, the seas, environment, and their own wellbeing. If, however, we as the current adults, don't give the children the information, they are left at the first post, only to flounder and learn by their own mistakes. As adults, it is far better for us, to pass on our learned knowledge, that we have learnt through our own mistakes than to re-invent the wheel for every generation!

CHAPTER NINE

YOUR BOY TEEN'S HEALTH AND INTO PUBERTY

All conceptions, in the early stages, start off as girls. Boys, from the embryonic stage, through development in the womb and then to birth, are different to girls. From about eight weeks within the pregnancy, a male baby's body produces the 'Y' chromosome, which then allows the developing foetus to produce testosterone. The production of testosterone makes a difference to how the body and brain develops in the male child. Testosterone production also encourages the penis and testicles to grow and develop. By the fifteenth week, both the penis and testicles are fully developed.

To keep the penis clean and healthy, the growing boy child will have erections while in the womb; this is a natural cleaning and healthy function for the organ. During pregnancy, and when the testes are formed, testosterone will continue to be made by the testes. At the time of the birth, the testosterone level within the baby's blood will be that of a twelve-to-thirteen-year-old, pubertal male.

Male babies need high levels of testosterone to allow their bodies to develop the male qualities needed to make boy babies.

After birth and by the age of three months, a baby's testosterone level will start to decline and will re-emerge by the age of four. At this age, it is his time of interest for cars, trucks, loud noises, running and jumping and being a typical boy. This testosterone rush will start to decline as he reaches five and settles down in time for school.

(From my own experience, with a baby boy, regardless of age, our son was always attracted to any form of engine, motor or building toys).

Testosterone starts to re-emerge between the ages of seven to eight years and in time for puberty. Having said that, some research is now suggesting hormonal development may take place earlier than has previously been stated. In a healthy child and into older male adulthood, testosterone will continue to be produced until death.

By comparison to girls, boys' brains grow slower and develop differently; boys usually catch up to girls by the age of eighteen years.

Your baby boy

When a baby boy is born, and like girls, the genital area of boys is in miniature. This is no surprise as all babies need time to grow and develop after birth. In boys, the penis is short and in proportion to their body size.

In an uncircumcised boy, the penis foreskin is left in place after birth. In a circumcised boy, the outer end of the foreskin is removed.

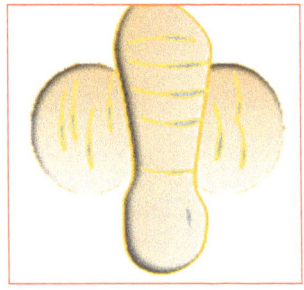

In this diagram, and at the birth of a baby boy, it can be seen how the foreskin of the penis is left in place. The scrotum, the skin's sack keeping the testes in place, may also appear larger and loose, keeping the testes safe. As the child grows and develops, the scrotum will tighten up until the time of puberty.

The hormone, testosterone is produced in the testes of the male and the ovaries of females. It is also produced in the adrenal glands of both females and males.

Testosterone is the main hormone in the male sperm supply. Sperm will start to be produced by the testes as the child enters puberty; and as said, *'it can be as early as seven to eight years, but may be earlier as some research suggest,'* but normally about eight!

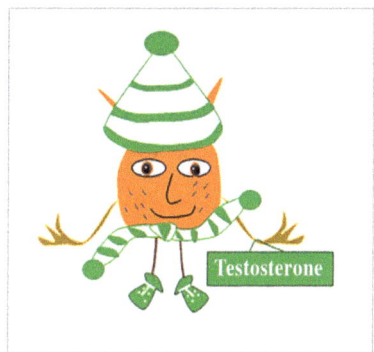

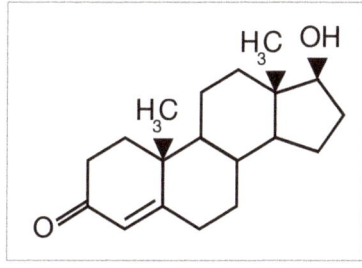

Testosterone chemical structure

As the boy grows, so too, does his genital area, this allows his body to function properly. During puberty and at different times, through the day and night, a pubertal male will experience different arousal levels from the penis. This is both healthy and natural.

Between these ages, the male might experience different and mild growth spurts, maybe some hair will appear on the body or in and round the genital area, and under the arms.

The scrotum will start to expand to allow the testes to do their work in making sperm, but the expansion also allows the testes to keep cool during hot weather, or if the body experiences excessive heat.

In this diagram, the scrotum is seen, dotted lines, and shows the expansion of the skin. As previously explained, this is a natural occurrence to keep the testes cool.

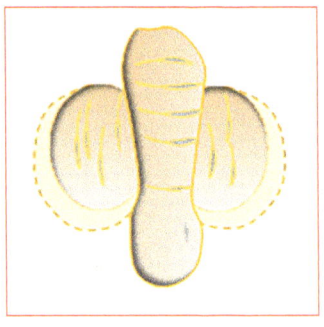

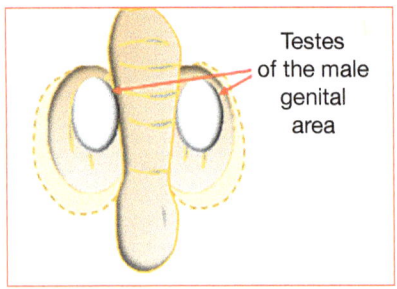

Testes of the male genital area

In a cool climate, if the testes experience cooling or coldness, the scrotum will tighten up.

Both loose and a tighter scrotum are made by nature for protection of the testes.

To allow the transference of sperm, the testes need to be connected to the penis through the vas deferens, a pair of tube-like structures linking the testes to the urethra.

The vas deferens transports mature sperm to the urethra in preparation for ejaculation.

Not all sperm go on the journey and leave the penis, some sperm die and are absorbed back into the body; this again, is a natural process that allows the body to make good use of what it has made.

For a child to be faced with all the processes of how its body works seems a bit premature, but this is the will of nature, nature takes over, this knowledge, in turn, protects your child and makes them ready for entering puberty.

So, what is sperm?'

Sperm is the smallest human cell. Each male makes many thousands of sperm every second, so there are a lot of sperm produced. In the below diagram, you can see the testicles and penis. There is nothing new or mysterious about the way the human body is made. It is indeed, a superbly developed design in human technology! So, let's look at how the male body works!

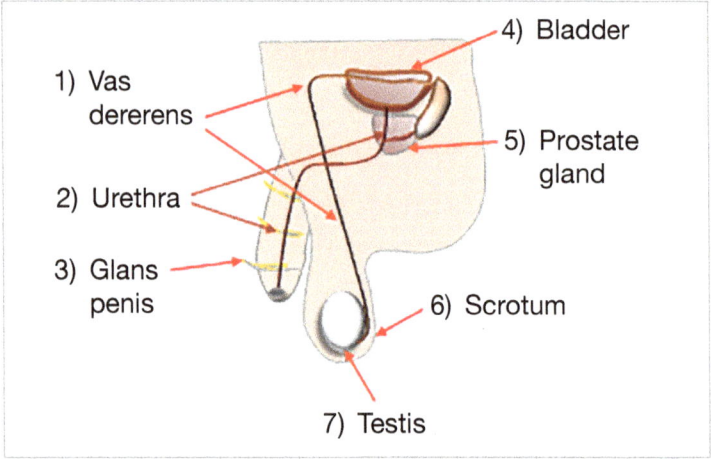

1) the vas deferens, is the tube that carries the sperm from the testes, number 7).

2) is the urethra, this is the tube that carries the urine; it is the waste from the fluids previously swallowed.

3) is the penis and known as a glans, organ, or member.

4) is the bladder and is where the urine is stored. We each know when we need to go to the bathroom, because we each get a twinge or message to our brain saying, *'you need to go to the bathroom!'*
5) is the prostate gland and this regulates sperm, when it travels up the vas deferens to the prostate gland, number 5). By the time the sperm reaches the prostate gland, it becomes tired. The prostate supplies much needed energy for the sperm to carry on its journey.

The energy supplied to the sperm by the prostate gland contains, carbohydrates in the form of sugar-based liquids including fructose, protein and catecholamines which include adrenaline, noradrenaline, and dopamine; these contribute to the hormone supply of the sperm. Once the sperm passes through the prostate, the sperm continues its journey and leaves the penis through ejaculation! This happens when the penis is in erection!

6) is the scrotum, as a male enters puberty, the scrotum, like the penis, grows, it might also go darker in colour.

The scrotum has the role to protect the testes and sperm, therefore, it is loose in the summer heat but will tighten up when the body gets cold.

7) The Testis
Each sperm carries complicated information

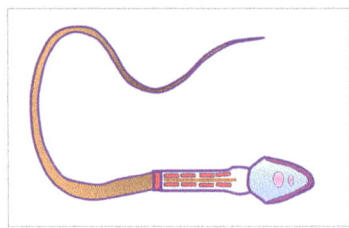

Sperm are made in the testes, and carry within its body and nucleus, information from our ancestors; that is vital information for the next generation to have.

For a penis to have an erection, there are many functions the body must perform.

The tissue and makeup of the male penis

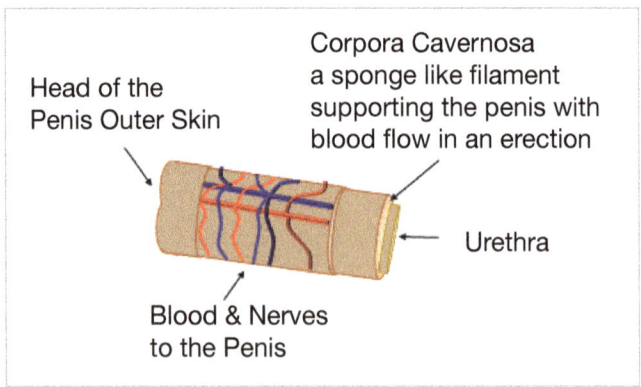

The head of the penis and the outer skin are seen in the previous image.

A penis, through the interaction within the brain, can receive messages from different areas within the body. Like females, the male responds through using their senses.

1) A MALE'S SENSES – include seeing, hearing, touching, words spoken, or through smell. Each of our senses have a direct link to the brain. Once received a message is sent to that part of the body that performs its action. In this instance, it is the penis. Depending on the circumstance, a male may respond to any of the above through having an erection.

2) NATURAL BODY REACTIONS – the penis can become erect through natural body reactions; it may also be described as an involuntary reaction. This is a message from the body to release or eject old sperm. This action is healthy, and the ejaculation of old sperm allows new sperm to be made.

As can be seen in the previous diagram, the penis is a complicated piece of human technology. It has an outer skin, a blood and nerve distribution network, and has a sponge like material that is made up in the corpora cavernosa. In an erection, the penis shaft fills: with blood allowing the penis to become erect. At the base of the penis is the urethra, this is the urine track that releases both urine and sperm.

Sperm always takes priority over urine and will be released before urine. This is all part of the clever human body technology that has been working for thousands of years and through many generations of the males in the world.

The sperm journey

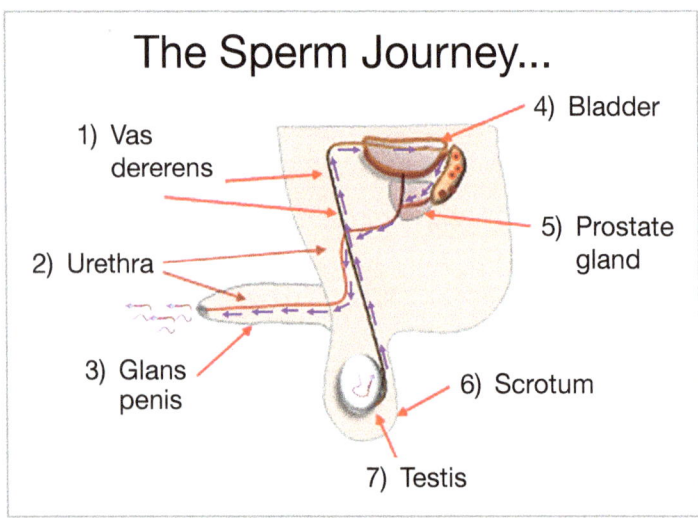

The Sperm Journey...
1) Vas dererens
2) Urethra
3) Glans penis
4) Bladder
5) Prostate gland
6) Scrotum
7) Testis

Sperm is not just a wet and sticky substance, it contains great amounts of information, which include the acrosome, mitochondria, and the nucleus, it also carries other information, but I am only speaking of the three just mentioned.

The acrosome carries enzymes which allows it to penetrate the female egg, the nucleus is in the direct head of the sperm, and it is this head that works within the female egg once fertilisation takes place!

Mitochondria contain a mixture of proteins and enzymes and your male's DNA. Of course, a sperm carries more information than that, it is also made up of organic molecules!'

As we work with our young males and give them the information about how their body is made and how it reacts, it will strengthen his awareness, add to his respect for his own body, and respect for his own future relationships.

A female body is made differently to a male body, and this is with good purpose, it is to create the next generation. By doing this, it ensures the future of the species, but, if in the act of sexual intercourse, respect for each other is lost, it can cause hurt, pain, humiliation, and sadness!'

KEEPING FOCUS AND EXPANDING ON THE INFORMATION

TESTOSTERONE – Both males and females produce testosterone in their bodies. Males produce more than females. The production of testosterone helps in both male and female health and wellbeing. It helps to stabilize moods and emotions.

THE SPERM JOURNEY – Not all sperm survive, and some never leave the scrotum. For sperm to be healthy, like so many parts of the human body and brain, including the hormones we all rely on, sperm needs to have a healthy and balanced diet fed to it from the food we eat. When the food eaten by the male lacks nutritional value, the sperm produced in the testes may suffer. Sperm is made off a complicated mixture of different chemicals which include, carbohydrates in the form of sugar-based liquids including fructose, protein and catecholamines which include the hormones of adrenaline, noradrenaline, and dopamine all of which contribute to the hormone supply of the sperm. Many activities, even in young males, can reduce sperm quality, some activities include drug taking, including vaping, alcohol consumption, obesity, and a poor diet of over-sugared, trans fat, processed food. Like all parts of the human body, sperm has a purpose, and if through neglect, poor lifestyle and activities, and personal choices, sperm is harmed or damaged, it will not perform as it was created to do!

THE 'HOW?' AND 'WHY?' – As the journey into adulthood continues, many young males will test out their environment. Testing may be by persuasion from their peers or from other young people of a similar age. High levels of testosterone may contribute to foolish actions taken. What our teens have not learnt is to think things through. To give you an example, many teens are impulsive and will act, then, if there is an accident they may fail to see, that the accident was their fault. Many will not understand that an accident is an unwanted outcome, and had sensibility been in their thinking, the accident may not have occurred. Added to this, is their lack of perception to the real dangers that they can place themselves in, is possibly not in their scope of thinking or vision, this learning comes back to past experiences, and our teens are still acquiring their experiences! When we experience a new learning, the brain puts down new neuron pathways, and where needed, synapses that help in the transference of information, including information about possible dangers in our pathway. Because the young brain of our teen is still developing and maturing, the necessary electronic pathways are not in place, therefore, many become susceptible to accidents and foolish behaviour!

CHAPTER TEN

THE COMPLEX JOURNEY INTO ADULTHOOD – AND AGAIN, THE VICTORIAN ATTITUDE

Having spoken so much about puberty, it is now time to bring it altogether.

Thankfully adolescence is now being recognised as a critical time in a young person's life. For many generations, young people travelled the distance and into puberty without any education or understanding of what was happening to their body, or indeed their brain!

And, to now marry hormones with puberty, and other life situations, that we may individually experience, makes a lot of sense.

It is not only puberty that hormones can make people go through disrupting times in their life! Other health conditions, brought on by hormone upheaval can turn a life upside down. And, of course, the sufferer, has little to no knowledge of why, they are behaving the way they are, or feeling the way they do! Life may become a complete mystery until the health condition or hormone disruption is identified!

Many females suffer with menopausal changes, some females are young when their body decides to change and some in their mid to middle fifties. Regardless of the age, hormones can go rogue, and leave us completely in the dark, because we have no idea of 'Why?' and 'How?' we are doing or saying the things we say or why they were said? The fact that our individual behaviour can, and maybe associated with how our hormones are working inside our body and brain, became a complete revelation to me!

I have spoken of the dual systems that can happen during puberty, but I think equally so, dual systems can happen at any age, because it is the hormones that are activated with different thoughts that activate our behaviour. Under different conditions, life experiences, and circumstance we each experience through life, we each, will behave differently!

The human brain
As a teacher, my aspiration for the respect, we should each give to our brain goes beyond any words I can

write on paper. It is the thoughts, held and coming from within the human brain, by certain people, such as scientists, that helped the world population to manage, though many good people died, the Covid pandemic. It is the enquiry and fascination of a subject that leads us to explore, investigate certain areas of human, animal, plant, and universal interest, that pushes human beings to ask more questions, and to seek more answers.

And so too, our young people, our teens are so similar in wanting to 'know more!'

Back to our Teens

I have spoken of brain development earlier in the book, and whilst, in the child, by the age of seven, the brain has developed, but is not mature until the age of about twenty-five. Science is now telling us, the human brain in our teens is still developing while puberty takes place.

Not only is the brain busily working to bring its working parts together, but the body of our teen is working in multiple growth expansion through many organ systems and major changes to the central nervous system (CNS). Accordingly, *'A dramatic spurt in brain development begins during adolescence and continues until the mid-20s, with marked development of both cortical and subcortical structures.'* (Goddings and others 2012).

Both the rapid development of the brain and body, heralds the changes within our teen's social network, relating to individualisation, and new peer-groups; this journey facilitates new progressions within their school friends or contacts, transitioning to further education or with acceptance into the workplace. As the progression of new beginnings happen in our teen's life, their commitment to family may fade!

This diminishing may shock close family members as the young adult takes on the world, and the world, they want to create for themselves. As we are aware, many young people, in their quest to find out about themselves, find they end up in trouble or in unsustainable relationships that encourage excessive drug and alcohol abuse and other destroying human values and human life.

Risk factors during adolescence

Many risks may be taken during the teen years and may be the results of early life experiences. Many risks taken may reinforce good or poor judgement or poor life pathways relating to individual wish lists. Having said that, many young teens become resilient and have a committed determination to meet their individual goals, especially if they face adversity within their childhood. As we have recently seen, the story of Sir Mo Farah[7], who at the age of nine years, became a victim of human slavery, taken from his home in Somaliland, to the United Kingdom to work as a child minder and had other domestic duties while imprisoned in his English home.

No child should be subject to abuse, but many are. It is the 'grit and determination' of everyone that makes a person determined to reach higher goals than they thought they could achieve, and remarkably, this all comes back to human thinking and attitude.

---

[7] British, long-distance runner, ten global world titles, four Olympic Gold and six World titles.

Human attitude

While at University, one of the greatest learning experiences I have had, was the day I learnt about human attitude. The lecturer said, and this was relating to teaching adults, *'Regardless of how hard you try, you cannot change another person's attitude unless they want to change!'*

How true were those words; they have never left me and still today, I take every above word and replay it in my head, and it is so very true. People must want to change, they must 'own' the changes they want to make, either in the way they think, behave, or in the habits they have created for themselves. If a person doesn't want to change, it is their right to stay as they are, and at times, it can be an extremely frustrating place, as an observer, watching people slowly destroy their life, health, marriage, or relationships because of the attitude they have adopted, and often, the negative habit they have, and the attitude they own!

Having said that, we can voice our opinion but as a person owns their attitude, and habit they have adopted, it is their right to keep it! If their actions and words do not break the law, they will stay within their 'locked in' world!

As parents we have a chance...!
You cannot bash a negative attitude out of your teen, but while they are still learning, you can come from positive perspectives if you see or hear a negative attitude developing.

Abusive relationships, bullying, racist comments, disrespect of other individuals, both people and animals, and a general lack of caring being shown for other people's beliefs, values, and ethnicity, can be modified if you have concerns.

One of the best ways to speak to your teen, is to sit down, face-to-face, and eyeball-to-eyeball and speak about exactly what is being heard or seen from their words spoken or actions taken. Do not speak as you do a job at the sink or while driving in the car, this is a serious conversation and needs to mark a changing point in your teen's life.

Executive control in the teen's brain

The brain, while developing has two functions within the long and shorter-range of connections within the neuron pathways working within the pre-frontal cortex.

Executive control within the brain is related to the maturing brain and the tasks our teens daily undertake from riding their bike, to working hard on their academic attainment, or playing in sport.

Because the executive control within the brain is still wiring, possibly re-wiring or making different or new connections with neuron pathways, some aspects of executive control may be less flexible, less automatic than when the teen is in their mid-twenties.

Because of the new neuron pathways and connections being put down over this period of a teen's life, in the learning, many teens have motor accidents! – It is the previously set down guidelines and working together that may save your teen's life!

Thus, during their mid-twenties, the neuron connections have had time to settle down, become integrated, and automatic muscle movement has become part of the knowledge within their muscle memory, and, or scope of thinking. This learning or the determination of learning is seen when our teen wants to learn to drive a motor vehicle.

Once executive control is established; learning new skills or behaviours can become challenging. If rewiring or the removal of bad habits are required, this task can be difficult.

Bad habits in attitude may include, little thought given to others with empathy and the human suffering they are enduring, the establishment of racist comments, the inability or not wanting to share or help another, the lack of understanding to minority groups, the lack of respect for females or males and their gender, regardless of circumstance, the persistence, and the inability to share, or see another point of view. There are other conditions that can be associated with what has just been spoken about, and this may need other professional, medical advice to understand the behaviour.

Therefore, if as an adult, you witness negative behavioural habits, a decline in personal value or worth, a lack of respect for other people, bullying of others, abusive behaviour to any other person, the situation needs to be brought into control by the observing adult.

The executive control, without early intervention, boundaries, guidelines, or limitations, may adopt bad habits which eventually form a negative attitude and indeed, could extend to the limited learning of new skills and positive behaviours.

Continuing with cognitive development of your teen

The human brain needs time and understanding to develop to its full capacity. Once we have a knowledge of the brain's systems and the need for the brain in both time and understanding to grow, and develop in our teen, both relationships between adult and teen can grow with exponential maturity.

Cognitive development incorporates the regulation of thought processes, actions and emotions which develop in the pre-frontal cortex. While the brain does its work, your teen will develop deductive reasoning, information processing, a capacity for abstract and multi-dimensional thinking, and a capacity to manage planning in hypothetical thinking, and realisation.

Sensitivity and peer influence

So many teens are sensitive to social media and the images or information found on those platforms. I have spoken about the dual systems within brain development, and the sometimes feeling of abandonment as our teens try to navigate their journey into adulthood.

Many times, and to add to the confusion, our teens will spend more time with their peers than possibly with the family. Accordingly, *'During the transition from childhood to adolescence, the amount of time spent with peers increases dramatically'* (Brown 2004) *'and peer and family values increasingly diverge'* (Gardner and Steinberg 2005; Steinberg 2008).

As some teens mature it is noted that some can become less susceptible to peer influence or actions given. Other research suggests, those teens who are resistant to peer influence have greater activity in the brain region that is involved in positive outcomes and emotional self-control. What this is suggesting, the sooner, our teens have the information about hormones, the way the brain and body work, and the self-knowledge to reflect on the words or actions they have taken, they can then modify their behaviour, in fact, take responsibility for their actions or words said.

Temporal discounting and consideration
Dopamine is a necessary hormone in the human body and brain; however, dopamine may be over manufactured in early adolescence, thus instant reaction or actions do not have considered outcomes, this is when our young teens get into trouble.

Under-age sex and intercourse – youth detention
Under-age sexual activity and intercourse is happening with many young people in Australia and around the world. First, it is against the law in many communities for teens to be committing to this pastime, and secondly, the young brain is susceptible to greater amounts of dopamine and adrenaline than is needed by the teen to live a normal teen life. The fact that testosterone and estrogen also play their roles in early sexual activity, can over-stimulate the brain which leads to a demise in school attainment.

I spoke earlier in the book about a young male who had been accused of rape; he was fourteen-to-fifteen at the time. Without any sex or puberty education, this male, together with the participating girls, had many girls eager to join in the fun. As I have said, like so many sweet journeys, they can end up with a bitter outcome!

After the accusation of rape, the young male appeared in court and is now spending his committed time in a youth detention centre.

The youth and participating females have possibly all suffered because of the lack of pubertal education and an understanding of how the body and brain work in unison. The brain being the obedient servant that it is, when the thought of sex and the pleasure received, if the females are willing participants, it would be difficult for the male to resist!

Had boundaries and guidelines been put into place through education and parental parameters, (talking face to face to the teen and given an understanding of the responsibilities of sex and intercourse), these teens would be aware, and may have taken note, of the responsibility of the acts before the participation took place.

Without education, we now have another young male in the prison system, with hurt and punishment caused to his family, and the families of the females caught up in the fraught activities!

Temporal discounting and consideration, continued

It appears that dopamine, in early adolescence, is over produced during the ages, fifteen-sixteen, affecting the pre-frontal cortex of the brain. Accordingly, *'the neurobiological basis for temporal discounting is related to developmental changes in dopamine activity'* (Pine and others 2010). Specifically, *'increases are evident in both dopaminergic connectivity to the prefrontal cortex'* (Kalsbeek and others 1988; Verney and others 1982) *'and the density of dopamine transporters'* (Spear 2000).

Therefore, and with current research, dopamine, and dopamine receptors, are overproduced in early adolescence, which would suggest, because of lifestyle, some in many affluent families, and a lack of pubertal education, our teens would be living with the notion, they discount the value of future rewards, without looking to long-term outcomes; this is in favour of having instant pleasure and individual sexual satisfaction, or instant gratification of the experiences received!

Without pubertal education, many teens will lack the guidelines needed, which will allow them to mentally balance the choices, or risks they take. They may commit to the following:

- Under-age sexual activities
- Under-age drinking and drug taking, including vaping
- Self-harm
- Low self-esteem
- Easily influenced by peers when peers give false or misleading information
- 'Follow the leader' rather than making informed personal, and independent choices and other actions that gets the teen into trouble.

Aggression and violent behaviours
Without guidelines in place, aggression and violence may show itself during the peaking, (fourteen to

sixteen years), of our teen's pubertal growth and into adulthood. Such behaviour can be seen:
- Sibling aggression.
- Spiteful comments and retaliation behaviour.
- An attitude, 'I'll get even' rather than thinking through the situation and the ability to ask, 'How?' and 'Why?' and the previously mentioned behaviours spoken about in the above.
- Lack of respect given to close family, and family members.
- Lack of respect for family values, traditions or culture and other areas of disrespect for the wider community.

Social media and your teen's perception
Over the last ten or so years, many researchers have focused on the intake of junk-food and the effects it has on the human brain. With social media ever pushing the ideal female shape, from enlarged female backsides, larger artificial female breasts, and smallish waists, there is also the 'flip side' to those images.

Eating disorders and dissatisfaction to a teen's natural weight can cause the teen anxiety and self-loathing, all contribute to the teen's emotions of not feeling 'good enough!'

Eating disorders and the lack of knowledge of food quality

The evidence is growing. Little do adults connect, hormones, behaviour and processed, over-sugared and trans-fats food, and the harmful ingredients put into many soft drinks including sodium benzoate. While sodium benzoate helps in general mould prevention in cleaning products, this chemical is found in many foods and some soft drinks! When combined with vitamin C, it produces benzene, a chemical known to cause cancer in humans.

Negative outcomes – the junk food diet

- **Memory loss,** when foods are high in saturated fats they hinder learning, add to memory, and verbal memory loss. Well known soft drinks were shown to negatively impact verbal memory. Having a sharp and heightened memory is vital to all students and young adults in learning.
- **Depression,** many foods contain additives, when consumed, the additives have shown to

alter neurological transmitters altering the way the human senses see and perceive food, food intake and the consumption of soft drinks. A dependency emerges, where the hormone ghrelin (a natural hormone alerting the brain to your teen's hunger at the right time for the body's need for food), once ghrelin is overridden by the chemicals in junk food, the body will continually want more food which leads to the onset of type two diabetes, obesity, and other health problems.

The need to eat more junk-food and artificially made foods and drinks leads to a vicious circle of want to lose weight while the brain is demanding more junk-food, which can lead to depression.

Artificial, synthetic ingredients now being put into everyday bought food and drink are contributing to depression and other mental illnesses in our teens.

> **Irritability**, and instant gratification of eating food on demand, (fast food), is the brain dominating our teen's inability to break the habit. The habit has established itself; the natural ghrelin release is now overridden by the

brain's demand for instant gratification, and the reward, is again, a meal of fast food and often accompanied, soft drink!

A regular diet of fast food can hamper the neurotransmitters, electronic signalling, (though not hungry), adding to the teen's dependency on instant junk-food, and in many instances weight gain, ill health, and lethargy.

Chemicals added to junk-food and drink, including multi-national brands, have shown to interfere with the natural dopamine and serotonin supply within the human body. Junk food intake may lead to irritability, a feeling of annoyance by the teen, short attention and attention to detail and a general feeling of being unwell.

I am now reinforcing information, once hormones are interfered with, through a constant diet of eaten junk food, and many poisonous food additives consumed, outcomes may be:

- Depression
- Irritability
- Dangerous thoughts, and

> Other negative ideas that can lead to serious health and wellbeing issues.

Research out of Canada, suggests, the nature of the fast-food market and indeed the advertising sent out to millions of people worldwide, is 'it's food on the run.' Julian House, Canada, *'Fast food allows people to fill their stomachs as quickly as possible and move on to other things. When you become used to instant gratification, you often find yourself becoming more impatient when things don't come quickly.'*

Over stimulation, hyperactivity – high sugar content – junk-food

It has taken many years of research, researching sugar, and yet, great quantities are consumed annually. In my book, 'Devils In Our Food', I have dedicated a whole chapter to this topic. Furthermore,

> We know for 'mouth feel,'[8] browning of the fast-food buns and the desire to 'want more' sugar is a vast quantity added ingredient. Sugar is also

---

[8] Mouth feel is the physical sensation felt in the mouth, on the tongue and roof. As an after sensation of swallowing, it is not related to taste.

added to accompany sauces supplied with the food order, thus, enhancing and adding to the 'mouth feel' by the customer and consumer.

Sugar suppresses dopamine, thus adding to many mood swings, mood fluctuations in our teens and other feelings of negativity relating to their wellbeing.

Sugar will only give instant energy that lasts a short time, that is why the actual food value of fast food is low in nutrition; it does not give long-term, sustainable energy! According to Cassie Bjork, RD, LD, founder of Healthy Simple Life, *'sugar can be even more addictive than cocaine.'*

We have seen much publicity about children with ADD, ADHD, both conditions may be linked to food additives, sugar, trans-fats, and other altered chemicals now used by food manufacturers in the everyday, worldwide food supply.

There appears to be a strong association between eating disorders, and fast-food consumption with pubertal teens. In a recent systematic review identified, *'advanced pubertal status or early pubertal timing as a risk factor for eating disorders or disordered eating in more than 40 studies in girls and more than 20 studies in boys. Early maturing girls and boys have higher risk of a range of eating disorders, including anorexia nervosa and bulimia nervosa, as well as symptoms of eating disorders, including dissatisfaction with body, weight, or shape.'* (Klump 2013).

A whole food diet

In a whole, natural, good food diet, the hormones are supplied with a positive fuel supply, and this allows them to work naturally. Eating a healthy diet contributes to stable behaviours and the 'feel good' factor.

A high-level energy organ

The brain is a high energy organ that requires great amounts of energy from the good food your teen eats.

The brain's demand for energy is about twenty percent of the food eaten. The brain's primary purpose, through electrical signalling running from the senses and through the body, is to process and transmit information. Wherein, some of the information is stored in both the long-term and short-term memories. All this processing, just like the computers we use daily, takes energy. The brain computer of your teen will not work if it doesn't have electricity or is flat and needs a recharge; equally, when our teens eat junk food, the electricity (food) from their diet, doesn't supply the brain with the energy it needs to run successfully!

Physical health and wellbeing
Puberty, and the association between puberty, physical illness, and hormone activation.

As the teen progresses into puberty, the activation of hormones, including the sex hormones, is heightened. Puberty, coincides with many autoimmune conditions, including the onset of juvenile type one diabetes. Other associated health conditions are asthma, various pain syndromes, stomach, and skeletal pain. Skeletal pain may be due to bone growth and expansion or juvenile arthritis. If you have concerns, please seek professional medical advice.

Secondary education and health intervention
During adolescence, it is a key time for adults to intervene and support their teen while they are educated in how to improve their health and wellbeing.

While the child is at kindergarten and up until about the age of seven years, parents maintain control of the child. As the child slowly grows and matures, then with the onset of puberty, the young adult will want to own how they think and behave. This ownership or demand for ownership may come early in the young teen's life; if this is so, sit down, again, eyeball-to-eyeball, with the young person, and talk things through. Please remember, the key to becoming a sustainable, and healthy person to live well, is to have boundaries and guide points in the teen's early life that will encourage respect, empathy, life values, and other important beliefs that contribute positively to the teen's longevity!

Secondary education
With an estimated forty-four percent of Australians (nearly half the population), not being able to read or write, this is a statistic you don't want your teen to be part of!

Early intervention in your teen's basic life-skill building is essential. If the teen has missed out on learning to read, write, or do basic mathematics, now is the time to stop, access, and help your teen in these areas.

There are many programmes now designed to do this basic learning. Having said that, it does not mean you sit your child in front of a screen and walk away, it means you support your child with the learning they do!

The dedication to your child's wellbeing, confidence, and self-esteem in supporting their learning, will be exponential with you by their side. It is a love of investment and their future security, as adults, that you are investing in, and a dedication of your time is needed to do this.

In my books 'Changes', it is with the investment of your time that you commit to learn and work with your teen that they learn about how their body and brain changes. The adult responsibilities that go with that change, and as a learning exercise, the teen, and adults in the family work together and as one unit.

From the World Bank (2006) research
During adolescence, teens make five decisions – pathway to adulthood:
1) Learning: Transition from primary to secondary schooling and from secondary to higher education

2) Work: Transition from education into workforce
3) Health: Transition to responsibility for own health
4) Family: Transition from family living to autonomy, marriage, and parenthood
5) Citizenship: Transition to responsible citizenship.

With your guidance in place and as our teens transition into adulthood, there will be displays of new behaviours, which exhibit responsibility and respect.

The Victorian shroud (attitude) – 'seen and not heard!'

The attitude of 'seen and not heard' is no longer needed, it is indeed, 'old-hat' and needs to be where it belongs, in the past!

Thankfully, as the populations of the world become better educated, and attitudes change, not only about puberty, but also the veils are lifted to outdated attitudes, worldwide girls and women, minority groups, First Nation people, people living with any form of disability, those living with discrimination or those people living in abusive or suppressive regimes will have the opportunity to grow and learn and become the person they were destined to be.

Adolescence and puberty are times of great individual human development and flexibility, and in some instances, risk taking.

Risk taking is part of each person's human development – some take more risk than others! However, with boundaries and guidelines in place, our teens will have the knowledge to keep themselves safe.

Understanding of the unique development, of not only the pubertal male, and female body, but how their brain, when given, positive information is their friend; however, when our teens don't take the time to listen to their intuition, and the knowledge they've learnt, can end up in many dangerous situations!

Collectively, individual, Victorian attitudes can and does put our teens in danger. It is far better to talk to our child in a safe and secure place than waiting or hoping the conversation will not be needed!

By the lack of education given during school lessons and sessions, the lack of parents openly talking about how the body works, all these components, help our young people to get into trouble. As, indeed, the young male now serving a term in a detention centre; this should not have happened in the twenty-first century. With education, he would have known his boundaries, limitations, and the fact that the law was broken by the acts of not only the male, but by the participating females.

Reactive education vs proactive education

In the case of the young male above and now his term in an Australian detention centre, supposedly, retribution for the wrongs he has committed, would come under the heading of reactive education. Some reactive education can be costly in human pain and heartache, and in the cost to the taxpayer to keep a person in detention when they could be at school or working, earning their living in the community! It's the same as closing the gate after the horse has bolted!' I would like to finish the book on a high note, by adults, including educators, taking the initiative and 'opening up' the conversation on hormone action and puberty changes, with proactive information given to our teens, a great deal of pain and heartache can be avoided!?

KEEPING FOCUS AND EXPANDING ON THE INFORMATION

THE HUMAN BRAIN – With so much said and the role the human brain plays in all of us, it makes sense for all education, at all levels, to draw into the curriculum objectives, the emphasis of working with and understanding of how the brain works when our children are in all learning environments. We have seen the transition from using nib pens and inkwells, to children or students, of a range of ages, using computers and tablets to do their learning, within the subjects, they are taught! Having said that, we seldom see or hear a teacher or educator relate to the brain of the child; 'why' is this topic, so far down the learning ladder that nobody mentions the absolute and most important part of human anatomy? If the brain doesn't work, nor does the child – it is a simple and effective equation to understand!

EARLY SEXUAL ACTIVITY – REACTIVE EDUCATION VS PROACTIVE EDUCATION – As with much of the information written into this book, there was always the mental 'tug-of-war' in the writing and research I did to bring this book together. As an author, researcher, teacher/educator, it was always my goal to give to my readers, proactive information, raising each person's awareness which allows the reader to collect informed information that will add to their skills-base, about the concerns they have, or the answers to the questions they seek! Therefore, proactive education builds insight, gives the 'switched-on' brain early information where decisive actions can be made, or informed comments said. I must admit, having taught, and counselled young offenders in the United Kingdom, taught sex education in Australia and then again, to see a young male caught up within the law and the outcomes he and his family are experiencing, did nothing but spur me on to write about, this unwritten about, subject! Every adult in the world knows about puberty, as they were too, once a pubertal adolescent! Having said that, how many of us have tied hormones to puberty? Not many I would imagine! It took my own learning with the inmates I counselled, the students in the schools I've taught, and then lastly, the real story of the young male now serving his time in a detention centre, to add the urgent need to produce this book, and now it is done.

The Victorian attitude of *'seen and not heard'* helps to support reactive education, this has no place in the twenty-first century

It is the intervention of knowledge that will guide your teen, in and through puberty safely, and that is what this book is about.

Thank you for taking the time to read such an important book, it will help to keep your teen safe,

Christine

References and acknowledgements

Research collected from peer-reviewed academic papers:

Bjork, Cassie, RD, LD, founder of Healthy Simple Life

Brown (2004)

Gardner and Steinberg (2005)

Goddings and others (2012)

Kalsbeek and others (1988)

Klump (2013)

Pine and others (2010)

Romeo (2010)

Spear (2000)

Steinberg (2005, 2008)

Verney and others (1982)

Viner and others (2012)

Whittle and others (2015)

Devils in Our Food and App also available at:
www.how2books.com.au

See
Devils In Our Food
For a full description of food additives.

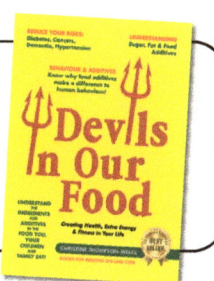

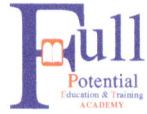

ONLINE SCHOOL PACKAGES

Full Potential Training offers a range of education packages. With our school packages for 'CHANGES', Children Growing Up, we cover the sensitive area of puberty and the changes that naturally occur in males and females. The story book at the beginning of each book allows the child to become familiar with the role that hormones play in making these body changes happen.

The packages meet both the Australian and United Kingdom objectives within Social Community Health and Relationship and Puberty education.

For more information, please email,

admin@fullpotentialtraining.com.au
Or, see our website, www.fullpotentialtraining.com.au

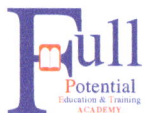

FAMILY PACKAGES

For many people, discussing puberty and the 'Changes' that take place within the human body are private discussions. They may not be easy discussions to have, but it is a necessary part of a parent's responsibility to their child or children.

For those people, we have developed Family Packages that include one book and a link that is the same as the School Package.

If this allows you to discuss this topic with your family in private, please contact,

admin@fullpotentialtraining.com.au
Or, see our website, www.fullpotentialtraining.com.au

www.ingramcontent.com/pod-product-compliance
Lightning Source LLC
Chambersburg PA
CBHW062034290426
44109CB00026B/2627